# A Professional Woman's Guide to Handling Stress

A Step-By-Step Process to Becoming More Productive

Hema Murty, PhD
Certified Personal Trainer (canfitpro)
Kettlebell (Kettlebell Training Academy) & TRX
Certified Yoga Instructor (Svyasa, India)
Precision Nutrition Level 1 Coach
Certified Spinning Instructor

ISBN: 1502338335
ISBN 13: 9781502338334
Library of Congress Control Number: **XXXXX (If applicable)**
LCCN Imprint Name: **City and State (If applicable**

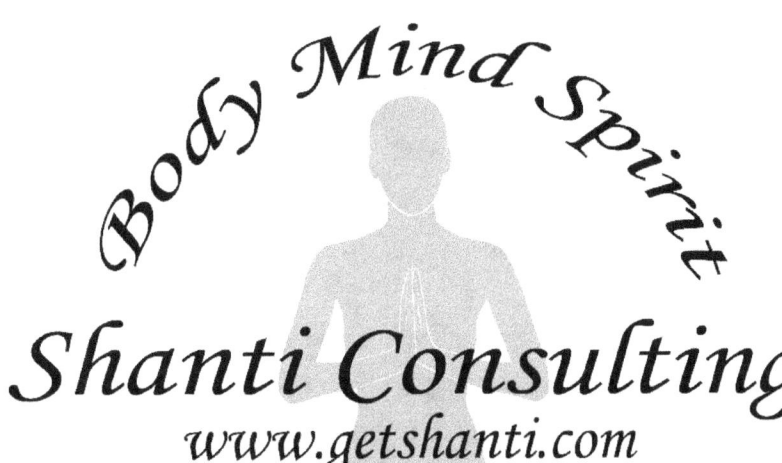

Shanti Consulting
www.getshanti.com

DEDICATION

TO ARDHANAREESWARA AND MY FAMILY

# TABLE OF CONTENTS

# Introduction

How many times have you started a "fitness" program? How long has it lasted? During the time you were dedicated to the program, did you see gains? Were they equal to the effort level of "fitting" your fitness program into your life?

Usually the first of the year rolls around. You make resolutions about your life. You assess the previous year and figure out the things you could do differently to improve your life. You're not alone. Basically, we all want to reduce stress in our lives. We get enough of it from all the things we actually have to do.

This book talks about our lives. It talks about the source of stress and how to keep it in check. We don't want stress to take over our lives. It is going to be there. It is a fact of life. In fact, it is said that some stress is good for us. If there are no project deadlines, then there is usually no project completion. We usually need some force behind us to prod us with that carrot stick. If company is coming on the weekend, then the house gets cleaned. If no one is coming, then more than likely the house doesn't get cleaned. Our plates are so full that forcing ourselves to put something extra on them is next to impossible.

Groceries get bought because we have to have dinner. We see our dentists because there is an *appointment*; otherwise, we would gladly put that off as well. Similarly, if there is something in your life that really needs to be rearranged, then you need an incentive, or the change is probably not going to take effect.

Let's take a look at fitness in our lives. Why do so many people start and then stop a fitness program? Life gets in the way! This is the simple answer. Now, let's take a look at how to keep fitness in our lives in a productive way. We have to take another look at what fitness means.

When we talk about fitness, we usually mean physical fitness. What we are missing is the fact that there is a body-mind-spirit connection that makes us who we are. Let's take a look at an example of this: If there is someone annoying you at work, don't you react with a headache, most times? Or perhaps the stress of the situation shows up in your neck and shoulders. Most absenteeism at work is owing to headaches, neck pain, shoulder pain, or back pain. This has a lot to do with how we sit at our desks, usually hunched over a computer. This sitting position, in itself, creates this list of physical stress. In addition, our mental anxiety from stress creates additional physical stress.

Breathing is a surefire way of determining how relaxed we are. When we are anxious, our breathing is shallow and short. When we are relaxed, we breathe more deeply, using our full lung capacity. Have you ever noticed how a baby breathes? A baby's breathing is full and totally relaxed. Watching babies breathe brings about real peace and relaxation. We start to empathize with their perspective of being in the moment; watching them, we forget about our adult life and think only about breathing. It is truly amazing. Isn't it true that we think better if we are calmer and less full of anxiety? Body, mind, and spirit act and react upon one another. It is possible to make body ailments go away with simple breathing; however, in order to make this breathing technique effective, it is important that we practice it regularly.

Therefore, this book is not about the next fitness program for your body. It is about establishing a body-mind-spirit way of life. The goal of this book is to teach you how to do things differently. Most of the ideas presented here are from my many years of training in the real world. East Indian philosophy is an attitude and approach to life. It is based on the teachings of the Patanjali Yoga Sutras and the Bhagavad Gita. Both sources emphasize an understanding of ourselves as the first ingredient in a productive life. This philosophy is used to present an attitude with which to create a better you, ready to take on the world in a more effective and peaceful way.

# Octopus Lifestyle

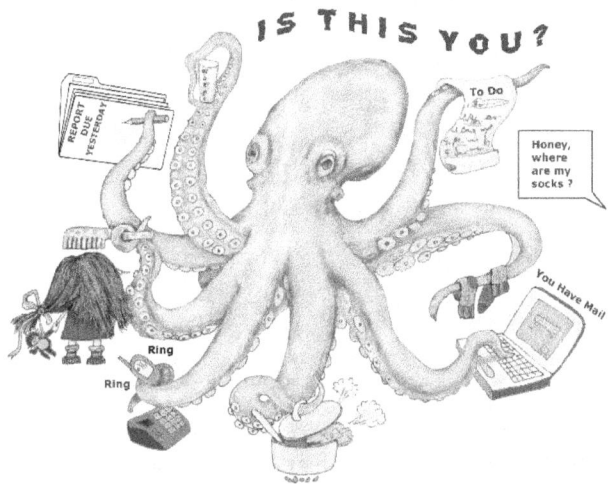

You are very busy. Trying to accomplish many equally important things at once is a fact of your life. As soon as you get up, your first thought might be about your family, job, or any of the other stressors in your life. You know you have to take care of yourself. Fitness should be a priority for you; however, real life seems to get in the way. Fitness is not just about the body. It is a body-mind-spirit combination. Your body acts on your mind, and your mind acts on your body. Then there is the third aspect of your being that is not body or mind. We will call it *spirit*. That side of you that gets the inspiration to do something in a unique way can be called spirit. That ingenuity that we all possess can be called spirit. Your body and mind act on the spirit, and your spirit acts on the body and mind. So your physical condition at any given point in time is just as much a function of how you feel and think as it is the physical fitness program that you are or are not following.

It is hard to ignore your family's needs in the morning. They will definitely remind you of their needs the moment you wake up. You get busy thinking about how to juggle all the stuff you have to get done today: *Wasn't that departmental strategic plan outline due yesterday? If only one of the managers wasn't away on assignment, I could have finished and submitted this report on time.* You quickly think of options to get around this. *Who is the second-in-command for that department?* This is usually when your four-year-old tugs on your pant leg. It looks like it was potty time a second ago. This is the now-or-never syndrome. If you don't clean up the mess now, it is going to smell like potty even during dinnertime! Of course, your son is now crying because his pants are wet. While you are in the middle of dealing with that, the phone rings. You notice the call display and realize that you have to answer it. It's your best friend who has been trying to reach you for days. If you don't make voice contact now, you might never know about her sudden marriage plans. You have been dying to know who, why, when, where, and how. Then you hear the computer notification: "You have mail." It is a vital e-mail from the corporate VP who is your ticket to that executive dream job. You are a heartbeat away from the job you have always been trying for. The VP is waiting for your response before he leaves the country forever on a corporate transfer. Your cell phone is ringing and it's your niece, who is living in Australia. You are her only confidante and advisor. Recently, however, you can never get hold of her and you have left ten messages on her voice mail, never hearing back…until now. *Is she okay?* you wonder. Suddenly your eyes fall on the to-do list for today. The list never goes away, and yesterday's stuff seems to be still on it. Your constant concern, which repeats like a tune you can't get out of your head, is *When can I make time for my workout?* Fitness schedules are usually the first to go because you feel healthy enough and it just doesn't seem like an emergency. But your physical, mental, and emotional depletion is just like that slow leak in your bathroom plumbing.

You can focus on only a few things at a time if you want to do them well. If you exceed your capacity, then you will feel overloaded and unable to cope. You would like to be at your best ability to perform. You would really like to do well at all the things that are on your plate. You know you can hammer out the best departmental strategic plan that the company has ever laid eyes on. Your talents finally can be utilized in the corporate suite. You know you can be a great mother to your son in potty training. You know you can be a terrific kindred spirit to your friend in need. You can be the best aunt on the planet to your niece, giving her good advice along the way. You can clean off that to-do list in a snap, and everyone will think you're wonder woman. You know that you *can* actually make time for your fitness schedule if you put your mind to it. Except that all these things come at once—not neatly one at a time. When stuff comes at you all at once, you feel the immediate need to respond to everything at once. You feel like you have eight hands. I call this "the Octopus Effect."

Your mental abilities determine how many things you can focus on at a time. Multitasking is also a function of habit. There are women who are used to running the whole family show, from a young age. They never miss a beat. They never feel that they need a time-out for good behavior. They never think of their own needs. They probably deserve a spa vacation! They look and feel great. Mental and physical fitness go hand in hand for them. Their body and mind walk the same talk. These women are solid. They have great faith in themselves. They are like the Rock of Gibraltar. Nothing takes them down because they have combined their body, mind, and spirit into an integrated, whole unit.

Are you ever going to escape the Octopus Effect? No. However, you can learn to deal with it in a more efficient way. It is not that stuff will one day stop coming at you all at once. It is that you will stay calm and relaxed, effortlessly. You remain unruffled in the face of challenges. The Octopus Effect has more to do with how you perceive and react to the outside world. The world is a busy place, and you are an active person with many demands on your time. That is not going to go away. However, you can train yourself to react in an effective manner to the demands on your time. The Octopus Effect happens when we try to do many things at once and get very emotionally distraught over the whole scenario. Are you at your best when this happens? Most likely you are not. This book will give many scenarios and training methods that will help to free you from the Octopus Effect. You can survive. You can be physically and mentally fit.

# Coping strategy 1    BREATHING

The easiest handle on your well-being is through your breath. Your breathing rate is fast when you are excited and slows down when you are relaxed mentally. Our goal is a relaxed, proactive view to life. To be effective, we have to slow our breathing down to reflect on the situation more clearly. Breathing has a tremendous effect on physical, mental, and spiritual health. Ultimately, we are physically sick because we breathe too fast. According to yoga theory, heart rate and body temperature are fallouts of our breathing rate. There is a direct correlation between our breathing rate and our physical health. Therefore, yoga theory states that we can improve our health by relaxing our breathing. As an example of the connection between our breathing and state of mind, consider how you feel when you are in the presence of someone who is unruffled and generally calm. His or her presence seems to send out positive vibrations, as if you've taken yourself to your "happy place."

According to yoga theory, everyone sends out vibrations at a certain level, and it is something you feel in their presence. Without digressing into the theory of yoga, we can certainly experience the tangible result of this transformation of our own vibrations. Loosely, "positive" vibrations emanate from our ability to experience a proactive calmness. This means that it is not the calmness of sleep, but rather a positive, "can-do" attitude without the anxiety associated with a nervous excitement concerning the end result. This nervous state of mind is more of the nature of "negative" vibrations.

In this sense, breath is the one reading we can use to determine how healthy we are. Our physical health depends on how our body gets its oxygen. The systems of the physical body depend on breath for their optimum performance. Therefore, it is important to get the pace of our breathing to correspond to our natural rhythm. Try the following exercise:

1. Sit with head, neck, and spine in one line.

2. Keep your hands in your lap.

3. Relax your shoulders.

4. Inhale and expand your stomach like a balloon on a four-second count.

5. Exhale and let your stomach go deep inside on a four-second count.

6. Repeat nine times.

7. Intermittently check your head, neck, and spine alignment and relax your shoulders.

Doing this exercise for thirty seconds during the morning rush will give you added energy to carry out your day's activities in a more effective way. You just have to take those thirty seconds. But it is worth it. It is like an energy investment to get you through the day. It is like refueling your car to get to where you want to go. You need to do it. Otherwise, you will be running on empty for all your day's events, and you will feel physically exhausted. You will not be giving your best to the outside world. When you have given the situation your best, there is a great feeling that comes from that, regardless of the outcome. That is where you want to be. You can be there during all the day's events; however, you need to practice your breathing skills in order to recall them when needed.

This breathing tool can be used during stressful events as well. Suppose you have an important meeting from which you are looking to gain a certain outcome. Think of that outcome. Then do the breathing exercise while keeping your mind on that outcome. Focus on yourself. Then enter the meeting room. You will feel a world of difference in your performance. You will also feel glad you're making the presentation as your authentic self, rather than as a nervous replica of the real you.

This breathing tool can also be used when you are working at your desk for long hours at a time. Take a breathing break. Your body will feel refreshed, and you will be more effective at the work you are doing. While working at a computer, try to relax your hand and arm muscles so as to be more effective on the work at hand. Relax the facial muscles as well. In addition, your neck and back are usually out of alignment while you busy yourself with finishing the progress report for that week owing to the standard "hunching" posture you adopt when you are under pressure to finish a task. To get yourself out of that mode, try taking breathing breaks to refresh yourself physically. You are more readily able to carry out your tasks in a more efficient and effective way.

We can try this same breathing technique in other scenarios. Have you ever given a party and felt it impossible to be relaxed? *Is there enough food on the table? Is everyone having a good time? Does everyone have someone to talk to?* The list of questions that race through your mind is endless. In the meantime, you are not enjoying the company of those whom you have invited to your house. Take thirty seconds during that event and breathe. See how much better you feel. You will also enjoy your own party more.

# Coping strategy 2    PRIORITIZING AND ESTABLISHING FOCUS

A useful technique is to prioritize and focus. You have many things that need to be done, but they can't all be done at once. You need to order your to-do list. Obviously, there are some things that really need to get done right away. It is important to address those first, one at a time. Focus on what you are doing at each task. This will relieve the pressure of stressing about items that need to be addressed later on. Forget about them for the time being. Instead, just focus on the task at hand.

The important thing in life is always your attitude. Your attitude determines everything. This is the secret. Sure, we all have our plates full to the brim—and then some. This is an acknowledged fact of life. There are many things you can do about this. First, you must focus on what is important. In the morning, the kids really need to be dressed, fed, and sent out the door on time. So temporarily ignore other items on your mental agenda. Don't let yourself think about them; it will only make you worried and send negative vibrations, as discussed in the previous section on the correlation between vibrations and breathing and effectiveness. You need to focus on loving your children when you are with them. This sends positive vibrations to you and your children. It creates a sense of harmony in your mind. Once they are taken care of, you then need to prioritize the demands of your day.

You must never neglect the care of yourself. You must make sure your nutritional and physical fitness needs are met. Otherwise there will not be a "you" who can take care of your family, career, and other things. Remember the example of the flight attendant who gives the instructions on oxygen masks: please put your mask on first before assisting your child. You need to be fit enough to serve the world around you in a way that will make you happy. It is about your expectations and not about the world's expectations.

# Coping strategy 3    WRITING THERAPY

A good way to establish priorities is to write. In the morning, you need to be clear about what you want to achieve that day. In fact, meetings will become more productive if you can first establish what you want out of the meeting. This requires thought. People go through life hoping all their issues will just turn out in their favor. Wrong. You need to know what you are contributing to the meeting and what you expect to gain from it. Being clear about these intentions sends these vibrations to the meeting. You will be more focused and definitely get something out of the meeting. In fact, your thinking about those ideas directs the energy during the meeting. As mentioned in the previous description about the connection between breathing, calmness, and "vibrations," your vibrations also direct positive or negative energy. This is what is meant by "directing the energy" in a situation. As your vibrations go, so does your energy.

The idea is to write your intentions in the morning. A minimum of three pages will help clarify your thoughts. Julia Cameron cited this exercise in her book *The Artist's Way*. You write about anything that is on your mind. If nothing comes to your mind, you write about your intentions for the day. What do you hope to expect from the day? Eventually other stories will come out, perhaps thoughts about people or situations. Write these down without any editorial. It is a free-form brainstorm. We normally experience stress and tension because of lack of mental clarity. These mental vortices then show up as physical issues such as headaches and backaches. Before you get to that state, you need to be clear about what is going on in your life. Sometimes we "shelve" stuff that happens in our life. That stuff is hiding, and we are fearful of it. This causes unexplained anxiety, which ultimately shows up in the body. Writing those three pages ferrets out the essential thoughts and worries in your mind. You do not need a separate, shiny new journal; you take scrap pieces of paper and write for three pages. Then you shred the pages. This is not something you reread. This is not something that is supposed to be beautiful. The point is to purge the stuff that is taking up space in your brain. Some days you may think you have nothing to say. On those mornings, start by saying you have nothing to say, and keep writing that until your mind will wander to what's really bugging you. Remember, sometimes you have to be patient for a long time, perhaps weeks or months, before your mind will admit it has something to say that you didn't want to face. But face it you must.

You can start writing by listing the things you hope to do that day. Even in this activity, be realistic and don't set yourself up for failure. Think of accomplishing a few things well and with low frustration rather than trying to do many things and finding out that you could not accomplish them. If this happens repeatedly each day, then we may get a sense of "failure" of not having accomplished what we set out to do. Personal experience has taught me that a person should strive to accomplish only one or two things a day. This relaxes the mind and body and enables a person to perform at a greater level. Those one or two things will be accomplished with full attention and pleasure. You will feel greater peace and a sense of accomplishment, and these feelings will serve as motivation for future behavior.

Having a to-do list is a great idea; however, it's easy to get overwhelmed by it and to allow it to become your boss. Stress increases, yet nothing on the list gets accomplished. The to-do list is a bookkeeping tool and nothing more. It cannot rule your life. You determine what you want to do. That is what you write down. Make sure you edit and update your to-do list. Sometimes you discover—even before you attempt to start the work—that items that seemed absolutely necessary are no longer required. For example, you may think it appropriate to contact a competitor to start a friendly relationship and create a better business environment; however, as you see that item on your list, you may get a different sense of what you need to do. Again, going to the idea of vibrations and energy, it may take us some time to get a reading of the energy level of a particular action. Is this action going to increase my energy, or will it be a drain? The calmer we are, the more accurate this reading will be. This sense can be termed "intuition." Your intuition needed some time to work. However, you would not have had that insight if you had not written down that action item on your list. You needed to see it with your eyes and let your brain feel out what that meant for you. Ramifications of an action are not always obvious. There is often the unseen factor. You receive an intuitive feeling that the action is not going to pan out in your favor. Be clear in your own mind about why you are doing something. It has to work for you. Don't do it without a reason. If something does not feel right as an action, it is not the right time for you to proceed.

A lot of authors and speakers have tried to describe this feeling of rightness as *flow*. If meditation, breathing, and yoga are practiced regularly, a daily feeling of living in flow is established. This flow can be achieved through awareness. This awareness can be gained and established by practicing the writing therapy that was described in this chapter. This simple technique is very powerful. You will be amazed at how your life can change when you try it. Many people get stuck thinking *I don't know what to write*, and their minds literally go blank when they sit down to do this, despite very good intentions. It is the actual writing exercise that is the therapy. If you *start*—even if you start by writing "I don't have anything to write"—you will get past this block. You could also start by writing your timetable for the day. This is also powerful. Many times we deceive ourselves as to time appropriation for tasks. We may have the day off and think of all the tasks we can get accomplished. However, because we had the day off, we may have started that day a lot later. So by the time breakfast is over, it may be a lot later in the day than usual. Then the computer syndrome hits, and after you have checked Facebook and Twitter and e-mail, you may be into the afternoon hours. So first, prepare a realistic plan of the day. Then you will not be disappointed, and you will have a more rewarding view of what you can get done in the hours you have. This time-allocating activity might lead you to be able to write out those three pages of thoughts. You may have thought of a person you had some interaction with that could have gone better. You can write about that. It is not supposed to be reread. It is not supposed to be kept for posterity. You will shred those three pages as soon as you are done writing them, so be brutally honest with yourself. If you really have "that guy was such a jerk" thoughts, better to confess on the page and let it out. Just write like you are telling someone. When you handwrite, the energy of the thought comes out of you better. The physical exertion of brain to hand to seeing it on the paper acts almost like a "flushing" system for that stuff that unnecessarily takes up space. Computers and keyboards are no good for this. We also know that nothing really gets permanently erased in cyberspace, so that stuff is still out there. Better to write it in longhand on paper and shred it immediately. This is therapeutic. However, like any activity, it will take time to get into it and reap the benefits. You must persist for at least six weeks to see the benefit. It may take you longer. Make it a ritual habit. Make sure you are alone and that no interfering thoughts can arise, from other people or the daily news. You must just sit with yourself and your thoughts. Bringing something relaxing to drink is a great idea. Most people do this exercise with their morning coffee.

Here's what we have covered so far in this Guide. We have three life-coping strategies: (1) Breathing, (2) Prioritizing and establishing focus, and (3) Writing therapy. Here's where physical fitness begins. No exercise plan will take root and make lasting changes until you have a handle on stress. High stress levels create chemicals in your body, literally undoing any physical benefit from fitness programs.

# Fitting In the Workout: What about the Real You?

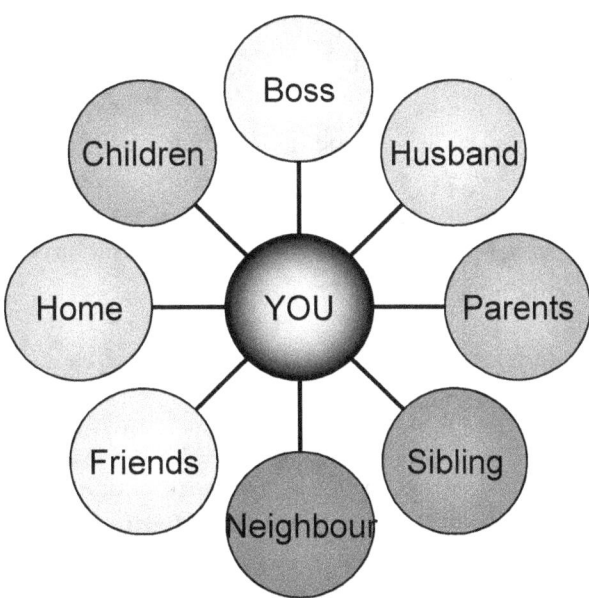

Where does physical fitness fit in when you decide that you are subject to many other factors in your life? Do you own your life? Or do you divide it up for everyone else to have a piece, leaving you to go to bed tired? From the moment you wake up in the morning to the time you go to bed at night, you are constantly consumed with satisfying someone else's needs—and sometimes, more than one person at a time. The diagram above illustrates your focus on your relationships and the way you dedicate your mental focus. Notice that there is no arrow to the relationship or needs requirements of YOU. But there is one connection to your ever-important boss, and the kids, and the husband. Aren't you the home maintenance designate? So, you pick up some cleaning solutions and some ant killer for the backyard, where you planted those awesome flowers only to find they became breakfast, lunch, and dinner for the ant army. Soap should do the trick. You spent hours on Google trying to figure this solution out, right? How much soap, and when to spray to be the most effective? All of this takes *time* to figure out!

Maybe your mother has been complaining about something recently. You need to check in on her and resolve that. Don't forget to keep in touch with your friends. They help keep your sanity, but then they can sometimes drive you crazy as well. What about your siblings? You want to see them…and then you don't want to see them. What about those neighbors who asked you to come over and talk to them about your fence and their bushes, which are creeping into your yard? Those bushes aren't ones you would have picked out for your home.

It seems that you are so used to externalizing that you are constantly looking outside for the definition of your life. It is an automatic reaction. You don't feed yourself enough with good vibrations. You look to the outside world to feed you with information constantly. You look to others to see what they are doing in their daily activities. What kind of clothes are they wearing? Where did they buy them? That's where you want to shop. If you don't, then you risk looking out of place. The social scene is dictated by the world outside. When do you make time to think about yourself?

For example, you may want to admit that you don't make yourself a priority. Then you have a place to start from; you can only go up from here. Start by looking at your wardrobe. Are you wearing the clothes that make *you* happy? What makes *you* happy? Many people who have a sense of confidence choose to wear something outrageous every so often, just because it makes them happy. They do this often enough for themselves. Their goal is not to attract attention; their goal is to tell themselves, "I am important to me. I don't care if an orange outfit is not what people would normally wear. I am wearing it today, and I am going to own up to it." You can also do this when going shopping. Give yourself permission to buy yourself something at least once a month. It should not be practical, like a toilet bowl cleaner. It should express who you are, like an indulgent body wash in your favorite scent, a colorful scarf, or another item of a personal nature. You can do this. Go for it. See how you feel.

Now look at what you eat. Do you eat what your neighbors eat? Do you eat what everyone at work thinks is great? Your friends at work bought blueberries from the farmer's wagon, so you better get those on the way home. It doesn't seem to matter to you that you don't like fruit that has been out on the street all day breathing carbon monoxide from passing cars. You must compare notes with your friend at work for the next day. Comparison is good to a point. If it is for information gathering, then it really does serve a purpose. You need to know which electrician does good work and is reliable and honest. Other people's experiences are a great data bank to get information from; however, comparison must be to a point. Comparison with others should be beneficial, it should inspire us to be better, and it should be limited. Don't live your life according to what others expect of you. Live it according to how you feel comfortable. You might take the time to imagine that other people are just pictures on a canvas that you made. Dream about yourself and what you would like to do. Do this at least once a week.

The ability to strike out on your own takes moral fiber. You need to know yourself and be comfortable with that definition. Are you happy knowing you? Are you happy understanding your own wants and feelings? What do you truly like? What makes you happy? All of this self-examination takes courage, because you have to be willing to face yourself. When you close your eyes and breathe, you are meeting yourself. For some, this is a terrifying prospect. They simply never want to take the time during the day to meet themselves. You have to wonder what they are afraid of. Are you one of these people? If so, try an experiment. Every day, for thirty days, get up in the morning and write down what you want. You can keep this information in a private journal. You can refer back to this list at the end of each year to review whether you want to keep the list or change it. You can also be proud if you have accomplished any items on the list.

When you write, phrase each thought in a positive way. For example, let's suppose you are not as eloquent as you would like to be when discussing topics with others. Perhaps you could write down a positive affirmation such as "I am successful at speaking to others." Seeing is believing, for our mental space. When you write down a statement, your eyes see it and transmit it to your mind through the medium of your hands writing it down. This kind of writing exercise is really an effective tool in getting where we want to go. This exercise makes our goals happen. Just believe that your affirmation will happen and be patient. You also have to be open to possibilities. Let your own thought space feed you for one bright, shining moment. This is one way to start opening up and letting yourself be comfortable with who you are. It takes courage, which we all have to some degree. We may need to take it out for a walk now and then, however.

The key to all of this is to be clear about who you are, where you are, and where you want to go. Then all of what you need comes up in front of your eyes. So how will you go about finding the real you? How will you know where you want to go? How will you know if you are there already?

# GETTING TO HAPPINESS

The first thing to ask is "Am I truly happy?" This question pertains to all the areas of your life, not just your work world. So many women tend to go to work and live a life that is on autopilot: We go to work to pay the bills. We don't look for satisfaction from work. Trust in the inner you to find that satisfaction without the fear of the outside world. We are all boxed in and shackled by the outside world's expectations of us. Something better is usually around the corner. You have to be willing to let go of a fixation on ideas you *think* might be right. That is where you need to do the hard work. It takes hard moral fiber to let go of the familiar and dive into the unfamiliar with faith that it will work out. If there are any doubts in your mind about the future, you need to clarify those doubts or face the consequences of this lack of clarity. You can't live life on autopilot for long. A turn will come somewhere, and you will be face-to-face with your fear. That is when most of us ask, "Is there a better way?" Suppose you did this prep work before D-day came. How much better off would you be?

A great way to find out what you need to make yourself happy in your current life is to write down your perfect life. List at least five things you would need to have happen that describe your perfect life. Where would you live? What would you be wearing? What is your typical day like? Are you married? What is your family like? What is your extended family like? Are you working outside the home? What are you doing? Be as specific as you can. The more specific you can be, the more it becomes a reality for your mind and the writing manufactures your vision. It is astonishing to think we have all manufactured the lives we lead by our own mental ideas about how our world should be. This is truly amazing. But we can then use that fact to get the life we really want. The important thing, however, is to rise to the occasion of being present for the faith ride home. If you have any doubts as to the reality of your dreams, then you still need to do prep work. Write down why you think there are obstacles to having this life happen. These are your fears. Look them straight in the eye and tell yourself you are not afraid. The unknown force is always around whether we acknowledge it or not. To be better off, however, acknowledging it is what you want to do. That faith in the unknown factor is what drives your dreams to reality. That faith works for you, not against you; however, you do have to let it work for you without interference. Don't doubt. The day doubt enters, brush it off like a mosquito that has landed on your blouse.

What about the real you? Are you a replica of the real you, walking around answering to every call of your name? Being unclear about who you are and thinking like you are unclear is going to make life very tough.

Instead, the way out is to find that real you. Do this by really practicing the writing exercises outlined in this chapter. Of course, we all hear that constant alarm of *But there's no time* going off. However, maybe you can press "Snooze" one day and luxuriate in doing just one exercise. Even if it means you start by writing down one line, it is a start. It will start the wheels turning in your brain, and soon torrents of ideas will flow from you. From that evolution of thought will come a firmer and better idea of who you really are and your wants—your authentic self. There, you will stand face-to-face with your authentic self and be in awe of that person who was in hiding all the time.

In fact, putting off writing is an excuse to put off meeting yourself. What are you afraid of? Aren't you curious to find out who you are and what makes you the person you are? Writing brings you face-to-face with who you are. There might be things inside your mind that are worth finding out about. Bring out the courage in you to move past your fear and start living life. I can't stress writing enough. It is a magnificent way to get out what you need to see and help you to move past it and make progress on all of your goals. This includes your physical and mental fitness goals.

## GETTING TO YOUR PHYSICAL FITNESS GOALS

Many people work out for many years yet see no changes in their physical fitness level. Some people who start a fitness program to drop some pounds are depressed that they don't see results. Let's investigate this situation and see what is actually happening here. The problem is usually an emotional block that prohibits them from dropping the weight they want to. They use the weight to cushion themselves against the world. If they did some form of writing therapy, then they might be able to drop the weight and move on. There would be great changes in their ability to breathe and store stress. We all store stress in our bodies, but it is not stored in the same spot for everyone. It usually finds a convenient place to hide and wreaks havoc on the person. Their fitness life is usually ruined. They usually gain weight and then develop more physical issues. It becomes a spiral nose dive into a danger zone.

If this is the case for you, what you need to do is open up. What are you afraid of? Write it down. Then prepare for the hardest exercise of your life. It is one that will open up your body and start you on your journey to health. Sit down with your paper and reflect on this:

1. Sit down in a quiet spot, undisturbed, for at least fifteen minutes or longer if you can.

2. Have a blank paper and a pen and perhaps a nice relaxing drink, preferably something like herbal tea.

3. Put your brave mind on. Look at your list of fears.

4. Pick something that is not serious (no life-threatening issues) and write out the opposite of each of those fears as if it was coming true.

Write your answers down in all honesty and then shred the paper. They are not to be reread. They are not to be used in the future. There should be no editorial comment from you during the writing session. Nothing is too unholy to write. It is all just life. It is what it is, and you have to face up to it. See if this exercise doesn't open something up for you. Do a breathing exercise right after you finish writing. Sit comfortably, close your eyes, and breathe in and out through your nose for one minute or so. Just let your mind float.

What else are you made of that you are holding back? You might find yourself to be a real explorer at heart. That part of you might have been hiding away somewhere. What does that discovery mean? It means that you will now find ways to express that explorer part of you in a more dramatic way. Perhaps that means real-world exploring, and soon your family will be having better vacations, exploring exciting parts of the world instead of the same old locations.

Perhaps it means finding a new part of your abilities that were untapped. Art, music, dance, or photography could be part of your fulfilled life. These undiscovered parts of you are what really cause you to be grumpy. You might fool yourself into thinking it is your husband's dirty socks on the floor or the kids leaving the light on in the bathroom, but really those things are just a cover-up for something deeper—something you were too afraid to face as part of the Real You. Once the real you gets out, however, there is no stopping you. Watch yourself shine.

# WRITING TO ESTABLISH THE REAL YOU

Writing should be carried out in the morning; however, owing to the morning time crunch with everything else going on, you can delegate it to another convenient time during the day. Get yourself some tea and a Do Not Disturb sign. You might want to get away to a coffee place or library where no one will bother you for a nice ten-minute stretch. Then write away. See yourself go places. At least give yourself a fighting chance to get your holistic fitness on track and relieve the hidden stress. A good cardio workout is a great antidote, but even that is only treating the symptomatic problem. Your stressors will reappear and cause physical pain again. Writing therapy helps you process stress. It makes things clearer for you. Where do you "file" people? Honestly, if people are not filed away in your mind according to their role in your life, then you are letting them dictate where your relationship goes. If you establish clarity in your mind, then you can be in charge of how the relationship unfolds. Otherwise, the energy of the fuzziness of the relationship is what directs it. This should not be. You are the director. You determine what role people play in your life. Remember this always. More importantly, remember it when you meet new people. The next time you do your writing exercise, determine what you feel each new person's role should be.

Fitness is not just about the body. That is where it starts. However, most people find they hit a wall in their workouts. A program that includes fitness of the body, mind, and spirit is what everyone should have in their week. This will ensure your physical fitness workouts are enhancing your fitness level and not just providing symptomatic relief.

# This Is Your Life

Each person whose needs we feel obligated to satisfy is actually draining energy from us.

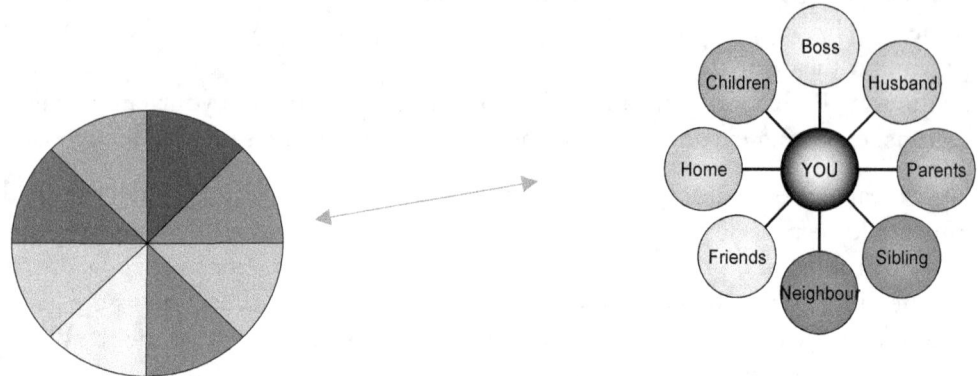

We start our day with a full cup of energy. Then, each time we worry about someone or something, we pour energy from our full cup into that person or situation. So you get up in the morning and start with a cup that's 100 percent full. Then your husband needs your help looking for his socks or shirt (−15 percent). You are down to 85 percent fuel already. Your children need you to get them ready and drive them to school (−20 percent). You are down to 65 percent fuel, and you haven't had your coffee yet. Then, you remember you have to go to the store on the way home to pick up dinner (−5 percent). Then, you remember you needed to get an item for gardening (−5 percent)—and the list of things to do goes on. You are down to 50 percent. Did you finish that presentation for your boss (−50 percent)? You now have 0 percent fuel left for dealing with traffic, getting yourself ready and to work on time, and anything else that comes up during the day. That is not much fuel to fight your way through the day, is it? There has to be a better way!

We need to feel more in control of our day so that we can preserve our energy for the important things we need to do. Looking for socks is not supposed to be energy-intensive work. It becomes so, however, because we are constantly gnashing our teeth while we are doing it. We are constantly draining away our energy thinking, *Why can't he find his own socks? Does he think I have nothing else to do?* Instead, the next time this happens, think, *Okay, let's just get this job done so I can move on. I can probably find these socks very quickly and keep the show running smoothly. It is also his way of communicating with me. Very different style than my own, but that's the way life is. I have a wonderful day full of wonderful things ahead of me. I am going to take this day to show the world how wonderful I really am. Let's get started.*

This scenario leaves you with much greater energy than when you started. It gives you the drive you need. Saying affirmations is also a wonderful therapy. We tend to go into a spiral nose dive of negativity. This need not be the case. It is hard work to speak affirmations and really mean them. But just say them a few times anyway. Say them twice with meaning. Affirmations do really work wonders, and they have a charm of their own. Who knows? Your brain might really believe them and make them come true. After all, they *are* true!

This really is *your* life. So what do you really want to do with it? You know you have a lot of great talents to give to the world. Are you going to spend your life putting those talents to good use? Or are you going to waste all that talent in useless complaints about everything? Life is for living. So figure out how you are going to live it and get started. The saying that we are not getting any younger has a lot of truth to it; however, we must not get fixated on age, either. We simply must be realistic. If we start getting worked up about age, it becomes another thing on which our minds are wasting energy.

# SURROUND YOURSELF WITH GOOD ENERGY

Another thing to note here is who we surround ourselves with. Our whole body- mind-spirit complex is vibrating at a certain frequency. We send out vibrations of the energy level of our body-mind-spirit complex. If we are thinking and focusing on certain aspects of life, then we will attract people who vibrate at a similar level. Similarly, we will pick up the vibrations of those around us. We interact with others who may be at different frequencies. When you interact with another person, there is an exchange of energy between the two body-mind-spirit complexes. Usually the less evolved person gains energy from the stronger person. That is why the stronger person feels drained when they speak with certain people. This one insight teaches us many things: We must vigilant and proactive about the people with whom we surround ourselves. If we must interact with weaker people, we must minimize the amount of time and energy that is spent in dealing with them. For example, we should not enter into arguments with them, because arguing is the best way to drain our energy right out. Arguing is an interesting dynamic communication concept. It definitely works among equals. But let's take, for example, a parent and a child. If you've ever had this type of exchange, then you can see the humor in the situation. Another way of illustrating this is as a well-informed person talking to a less-informed person. The basis for argumentation is lacking; it can degenerate into an emotional exchange.

There are several different energy vibrations that can be classified into three broad categories. These categories were discovered by early advanced people about seven thousand years ago. This body of knowledge was orally transmitted until it was written down about one thousand years ago. The lowest level is called *tamas*. The middle level is called *rajas*, and the highest level is called *sattva*. These are Sanskrit words that do not have a good English translation; however, we can describe the effects of these categories. For example, tamas is characterized by dullness. Think of an animal that goes on instinct and doesn't "think." That's why so many animals end up dead on the road. Dogs don't usually think; they just act or react. Rajas is characterized by acquisition of money, power, fame, or other worldly motivations. Sattva is characterized by a higher motivation like truth, ultimate goodness for the world, and peace.

We are usually a combination of all three; however, some people are more predominantly one or another. If someone who is predominantly sattva is having an argument with someone who is predominantly tamas, then what is going to happen? First of all, nothing constructive can take place because it is like the two people are speaking different languages to each other. There will be frustration and anger from the tamas person, and the sattva person will feel an energy drain and the impulse that he or she must refuel. The sattva person has to constantly refuel, or his or her energy drains can be significant. It is the price you pay for being more evolved. Basically a more evolved person is there to help the world with his or her advanced understanding of how the world works. More importantly, the sattva person knows how we interact with the world.

This shows you how important it really is to surround yourself with the right people and minimize your interaction with those who are at different vibrations than you. The times to watch are when you feel beaten by the world and circumstances around you. This is usually when you slip. You start your descent into lower levels of behavior. You make friends with people who really don't help you but instead prey on you. This takes your energy level further down. Then, there is the possibility of staying at a lower level of vibration and attracting those types of negative energy-draining people in your life. Instead, you must rise during adverse circumstances. You must strive to be alone or lift yourself higher to surround yourself with strong people, if even for short time. Such people do exist in the world. You must pray to be led to them. They are not around the corner waiting for you. They must be sought. A yearning soul will find them and be led to the proper path to rise above the vagaries of the world. It is at this time that you are the most susceptible to being taken advantage of. This is when you need to be the most careful. Help is never far; however, it must be sought deliberately.

You see many examples of disparate character types in daily life. Sometimes you are explaining something to someone who you usually consider intelligent; however, you find during the course of the explanation that nothing you say is getting through to him or her. It is as if you are both speaking different languages, even though you are both speaking English. This is because your frequencies of behavior and personality are radically different. At this point, you must become aware of the fact that you are not on the same wavelength as the person you are talking to. You must stop wasting your energy in further explanation. It is draining you. Being aware of this aspect of human personality is very important. It helps prevent energy drains.

We learn to avoid having extensive interactions with some people. It is a useless exercise and leaves us depleted. Instead, we focus on people who are more at our level of vibration. When we learn to do that, we need not seek out those people; they are attracted by our awareness, and they come to us. It is an automatic reaction. Awareness brings about circumstances to better display that awareness. If we are aware of spirituality, spiritual people come to our circle.

There are others whom we must avoid. These are the "fakers." These are people who know they should be better and realize they are actually very low. When they meet more-evolved people, they fake that they are also more evolved and speak of spirituality. This is actually more dangerous than those who are ignorant and full of tamas. Seeing through these people takes a little more work, but it is not hard because they give themselves away.

To illustrate this point, here is an anecdote. I once tried to set up a session with a "spiritual" coach who advertised herself as such. After we had set up the appointment, I had a family issue that required me to reschedule. When I tried to explain this to the "coach," she got incredibly angry. "Hmmm" is what I thought of that. Even if I had inconvenienced her, I doubt that it is good business relations to show it, especially if your business is to be a "spiritual coach."

In the same way, we must always be mentally alert for those who wish to steal our fire. There are those who are jealous of our well-adjusted mentality and seek to try to take us down. We must, however, focus on ourselves and uplift our own inner light. Then we must focus on surrounding ourselves with those who can preserve and uplift our spirituality. Remember that it is good to help people but not at the expense of our own energy. Also remember that we are here to evolve. All the things of the world are here to aid in our evolution. We must not be taken in by them as the be-all and end-all of life. In fact, they are just here to see what we are going to do with them. Living is a twenty-four-hour-a-day, seven-day-a-week job. Don't let your guard down. Be aware that no one is here to help gratis. Everyone has an agenda. We need to build up our own strength in order to survive.

It is important that everyone strives to maintain his or her energy levels without being diminished by negativity. To do this, it is vital to take stock. Where are you? Where do you want to be? Which people give you energy? Which people drain your energy? Formulate a map so that you can minimize the drainers in your life. Make sure you spend more time with those who have energy to give.

# Emotional Drains

We need to realize that we are not the sum of our relationships. In other words, who we are is not defined by our relationships to others and how we react to them. Otherwise, it would imply that we constantly need to do something with others in order to be who we are to satisfy that definition. Then you would be a human *doing* instead of a human *being*. However, if you centered yourself in your sense of being, you could still relate to everyone, but it would be as someone centered in herself and establishing relationships with others.

This method does not deplete energy. You are centered in yourself. Taking care of you becomes job number one, and you can then relate to others from a more wholesome standpoint. You will notice what a big difference this makes in your mental balance. You will feel more relaxed and have time and energy to focus on your own well-being.

Anytime you devote emotion to any thought, it represents an energy drain. You have let someone else take the reins, and you are susceptible to the way in which that person would choose to emotionally manipulate you. You are then at his or her mercy. If, however, there are no energy links or outlays, your total energy is available for looking at you and establishing your relationship with others. You need to be clear on what defines "the real me." You can go back to the centered approach of focusing your attention on your relationships with others, centered from you and not from what they think your relationship is.

This is the secret of retaining the energy of our being within a more harmonious definition of who we are. We will feel better about everything, especially ourselves. Our problems with the world emanate from our identification with the wrong description of us. We need to be clear and stand balanced in ourselves. Then we can move around from a position of strength. We find this metaphor often used in hatha yoga. For each asana, or posture, we realign our balance with breathing and refocus ourselves within us. From this position of balance, we can move around to our next posture. We will look at this connection with yoga in a later chapter on methods of gaining balance in life.

Our usual perception of ourselves is unrealistically self-deprecating. We also surround ourselves with people who have equally low opinions of themselves. This gives our own view validity, and we enter into a spiral nose dive. We wonder why nothing ever changes in our lives.

In actual fact, we need to change this around. The man on the white horse or the hero will arrive in our lives when we are ready to receive them. We must not look like we need them to bring us up. We need to bring ourselves up first. How do we go about doing this? We must first look at who is around us in our life— who takes us higher and who takes us lower. Make a private list. You need not share this with anyone. You can even shred the list once you understand the scenario of your life. You simply need to visually see how your life is set up for further failure instead of improvement. Don't get rid of friends. That is not the answer to this. Also, you can't get rid of family members. This exercise simply makes you realize where your energy is going and being wasted.

If you want to turn your life around, you need to change the landscape. Minimize the time you waste with people who are energy drains. More importantly, during the time you spend with them, be detached. What does this mean? It means that during the time you are with them, you refrain from identifying yourself with them. You are two separate people leading two separate lives. You are interacting at some level, perhaps in a conversation or an activity like shopping, but that activity does not entitle the other person to a piece of your energy. Simply share space, but keep your mind to yourself.

It is a guaranteed fact of life that some people around you will try to bring you down. Hold your ground. Observe rather than be taken in. Listen but don't react. Pretend what you are seeing and hearing is a nice story about a personality—like a character in a book you are reading—that is unfolding before you. This kind of detached observation can be quite humorous. I was once having lunch with a woman who seemed well adjusted. She was helping me in a business transaction that would result in no monetary gain for her; therefore, I wanted to take her out to lunch. At one point in the conversation we were discussing a third party and their policies. I was relating their point of view, and she objected to it. In the middle of the conversation, she burst into anger. I then reminded her that I was simply relating a point of view. At this point, she said, "So I needn't get all hot and bothered by it?" I replied, "You needn't get all hot and bothered by anything." I really didn't understand what was going on until I reviewed it later. Her anger was a volcanic eruption of the events in her life. She never gives herself permission to fume; therefore, she finds something wrong somewhere and then lets her negative feelings out. The object of her anger is probably not what she thinks it is. She is upset over her own personal circumstances. In fact, she is a walking powder keg. I now refrain from spending any time with her alone or communicating with her at any great length.

Being aware of powder kegs is a learned technique. In fact, consider that most people operate with anger that way. Their neuroses are usually unresolved. They are angry and don't find ways to vent. Venting should be a constructive daily exercise. If you don't vent, you cannot become holistic in your view of the world. If you find those around you constantly telling you of their problems, and weighing every conversation down, then it is a sure sign to leave them out of your inner circle. Their grumblings about the world will only sap energy from you.

After distancing yourself from negative people, you are faced with the question of how to fill the void that is left for positive company. That company will come. Don't be in a hurry to fill that void. Fill it with your own company in the intermediacy. Pray that the right companion will come—someone to help you in your life and also someone to whom you can be of help. This is a symbiotic relationship where both people gain. Being with yourself is actually a very deep bonding experience. This is the first relationship that you must establish. Make dates with yourself. Go to the museum, art gallery, library, and even the movie theater. These are great dates. Live for a time with yourself. Eventually, when you establish that relationship with yourself, someone else will come along that will add to your strength and not decrease it. But be on guard and observe. Partnering with people is a crutch. Learn to go it alone. Then the right solution will arrive for you.

Another way to ensure that is going to happen is to write. Spend time writing a list of the attributes of the person you wish to be with. Look at it every day. Dream about that person and how you would spend time together. How would you feel? Make that a reality for yourself. Then go about each week spending an hour in a place where you think such a person would show up. Spend that hour constructively while you are on the lookout. During that time, mentally tell yourself that person is here or will arrive. Mentally review the attributes of that person. Mentally review how you would feel and act out a scene that might happen. Spend that hour in the place you think that person would be. You also need to be patient. Being anxious is a sign of fear. We must get rid of fear if we want to make progress in our life. Fear is what drags out those ugly monsters with which we previously surrounded ourselves. They wait for the weak moment and sap our strength. Throw fear away. Instead substitute the love of this person who is going to enter your life. Make way for that person.

Let's consider an example. Suppose you want to meet someone who has the following attributes in your list. Only a small portion of your complete list will be shown here:

1.  Intelligent

2.  Handsome

3.  Interested in music

4.  Good conversationalist

5.  Handy around the house

So where would you go to meet such a person? One thing to note is there is never a dearth of places to go to meet people. There are many places to go, most of which you could probably not exhaust. If you want intelligence, then you might start with activities of an intellectual nature. Have you considered a poetry reading? Art galleries are great. You may want to sign up for a tour, which might attract such a person as well. We really can't say anything much about the handsome part. There are handsome people in every realm of life. "Interested in music" is a very general statement. You would need to narrow that down to what type of music.

I was once coaching a lady who wanted a friend who was interested in music. The problem with that client was that she read too many self-help books. She was getting too many conflicting messages from these books and became unclear on what to do, specifically. You must be focused in life. You must join your head to your heart. When you take in information, don't take it in from all sources. There are many people in the world who want you to listen to them. You need to check out their credentials. What gives these people the authority to dole out information? My client was reading everything and listening to everyone. She was appearing desperate, even to herself. This is where the problem begins. If you seem desperate to yourself, then it is a sign of fear. Let it go. Live with the fact that you are here for you, and get to know yourself. This same woman **was crazy about skiing. She m**et a friend who did not ski and was unwilling to learn. This was a recipe for disaster. Red lights should have gone on for her; she needed to give herself more respect than to hang around with someone who was not willing to share in her enthusiasm for something that was really a part of her.

The authentic you should never take a backseat. If you find it doing so, then you must reevaluate. In the case of my friend, she really needed to focus on the ski parties and other social events. She needed to crack herself out of the "fear casing" she had built.

Fear should be tossed away like an apple core. It is totally useless and just takes up space. Be authentic to yourself and identify your needs. Then try and see how you can fulfill each one. If you have a family problem and you are bitter about it, then you need to write that out. Every day, that writing therapy should take a half hour, minimum. Write away your angst against the world. Get comfortable with the hand life has dealt you, and make something of it. I know a woman who was born into great circumstances but by fate got married into a disaster. She grew stronger from it and was always happy. On the other hand, I know a man who had it made after marriage yet was miserable all his life. In fact, he created misery for everyone around him.

The emotional drains are the things to watch for. Never let your guard down with others. That is why setting aside time to be alone and reenergize is important. During the time you spend in solitude, you can let your guard down and relax. Let your hair down. Get comfortable and vent all you want. Make room for something better when you do that.

# Define Your Sense of Being

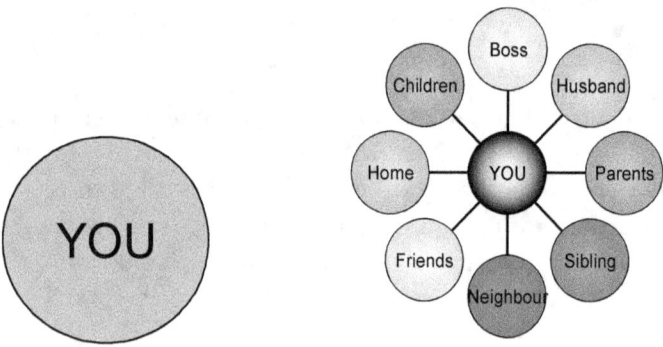

You are still you, without those ties to others through relationships. In fact, you are a better you, because your self-definition is based on something internal to you, rather than external relationships. Those relationships, in which you are constantly serving others' needs, or their expectations of you, drain you. Instead, reestablish the connection with yourself. You should dream of yourself as a complete person, independent of others. This is the reality, and when you dream of it, you will be even closer to that reality. Eventually, you will prove to yourself that your relationships don't define you. Your inner sense of being defines you. What will be different is your perspective on your relationships. Those relationships will be better when you approach them from the strength of your inner sense of being. This attitudinal shift delivers an air of confidence. Others can sense that feeling of strength. They may not realize what the source is or really be certain of what it is that is inspiring them. Your presence itself will inspire people.

You are a more honest, authentic you without your relationships defining you. Your *honest self* shines forth, and if you approach people from that vantage of strength, you will be better able to deal with the relationships.

Therefore, without all the links of relationships, we hear a resounding "YES" in answer to the question "Am I still me?" We realize that all those outside requirements and energy drains no longer gulp our energy up. We are constantly feeling energized.

Let's consider an everyday example. You walk into a room full of people, mostly male, who are in a supervisory position to you. Your heart begins to flutter. Your well-crafted presentation suddenly collapses when you open your mouth to begin to speak. Where are you? Where is your mind? Your mind is nowhere near your presentation. It is hovering over and replaying the question *What if they don't like me or what I say?* In spending all your energy supporting that hover formation, you lack any focus on why you are in that room in the first place. At this point, your body has taken the emergency response cues from your mental drill. Your heart is beating faster and you are nowhere near calm. An extreme level of anxiety would better describe your state of being at that time.

The best way to retrieve the real you from that zombie state of nonfunctional being is to focus. If you use your body as a tool, you can refocus your mind and get the job done efficiently. Start by regular breathing. Do this for a minute. By this time, you have retrieved your mind from its anxious hover zone and returned it to the here and now. You suddenly remember that you are here to educate people using your presentation. You are passing on knowledge that only you have because you did the work for the presentation. You are here for a purpose. Remember that. You are important only to you. If others are listening and gaining from that, you are the richer. However, it is important for us all to remember what purpose we are serving in the grander picture. If you are appointed to give a presentation, then use that opportunity to educate. What do you know that others don't? This is the best place to start. You will serve a need with this attitude. The people's appraisal of you does not enter into this equation. For what reason would you include it as part of the scene?

At this calmer state, you can serve the purpose for which you are there. In addition, you have much more energy to serve yourself. Your delivery will be more efficient. Your audience will understand you at a level deeper than words. This is because you are delivering your message with more than just words. This extra dimension comes from the ability to separate yourself from the emotional world and focus on a world in which you serve humanity. This is a better vantage point from which to communicate with someone.

In a previous chapter, we discussed difficulty in communication with those people who are at a different vibration than ourselves. As well, sometimes there is an underlying fear that we sense. Women generally have very good intuition. Sometimes we sense fear when talking with someone. Thus, communication gets blocked. People get frustrated with each other. Ultimately they just label each other as difficult to get along with, but nothing is further from the truth. We are all beautiful, and communication can be beautiful, yet sometimes our fear gets in the way and we turn ourselves into frustrated beings. Anger is always a façade for fear. Is it easier to face fear? No. But identifying it is a step toward solving the problem. At least you know it's there. Ignorance is not bliss. Knowing a fear exists enables us to reach out to dispel it. Why do we get attached to some people? Why do we feel that the world is empty without a certain person? Is it really true? Or are we just afraid to face the world alone? The point is that we are not alone, although it can be difficult to believe that.

Spirituality is about believing in yourself because you are more than what you see as a body and mind combination. The human spirit, or inspiration, is a great force. Left buried in most of us, it is a hidden treasure. To uncover it, you just have to start thinking about it. Perhaps during your morning writing exercises, you can ask the question about how to tap into this spirituality on the page and let your mind think about it. Synchronicity might bring forward someone who can help you. This is how we survive.

How would you alleviate the feeling that it's you against the world? You could tell yourself that we are all in this together—and the truth is *we are*. It is never you against me, or us against them. It is all of us in the universe together. We are all working toward our ultimate freedom. We have to evolve by feeling a sense of oneness. Life is a journey taken by you as you discover your relationship to the universe. Sometimes it is a journey you feel alone on; you may feel a personal God will help you through this. Develop that aspect of your life. The journey of life is just like going to school. Your parent may take you there, but it is up to you to actually attend the classes and learn. You also have to figure out how to learn on your own and how to get along with other people in order to survive.

Hey, does this sound a little familiar? Isn't this what we do every day as adults? We don't have a clear-cut teacher and classroom, but we do have a "teacher" figure of authority. We have colleagues who work with us in the gigantic classroom, which now includes everyone we know. The lesson never ends. It goes on all day, and you can have many teachers.

The moment you realize that the world around you is a reflection of you is the same moment in which you finally start on your journey to happiness. It's a common tendency to want to blame everyone outside: "The boss is out to get me." Is this something you hear yourself saying? Then now is the time to turn your life around and stop going down that spiral nose dive toward more and more failure. If you ever feel that the boss is out to get you, then in reality, you are out to get yourself. You don't want to be there. You feel something is lacking in your performance. It's easy to turn your fear around so it comes out of the boss's mouth. While there are some people with whom it takes a monumental effort to maintain a relationship, you need to examine where the negative energy is coming from. How much of it is your doing? Do you hold preconceived notions of yourself, of the boss? Examine this first. The boss is a perfect reflection of how you want him or her to be. So how do you turn your picture of the boss as the devil incarnate into a picture of someone with whom you establish a positive relationship?

This activity is the key to life: Take time out right now and make a list of all the things you both have in common. Read it over to yourself. Read it over every morning. Focus on that. The next time you see your boss do something that makes you think he or she is out to get you, focus on some item on that list. Keep it in your purse or wallet if you want. Reinforce the positive. This is a positive strategy for turning things around for you both.

We need to focus on the positive between ourselves and the world around us. Our outside world is a reflection of our inner world. This is the secret of life. If you feel something out there is not right, then focus on what inside you is not right. Let's look at an example: a woman thought she had no friends. It was not that she was not a social butterfly; on the contrary, she was seen everywhere. She was attractive and had a great personality. She made friends easily; however, she always kept them at arm's length. Upon my investigation it was found that she harbored resentment toward most people. She thought she was beyond them and superior to them. In fact, she was very well accomplished and didn't suffer fools gladly. It was really a fact that most people couldn't hold a candle to her. She was intellectually very much beyond most people's capacity to think. It was clear to her that she would not be able to find many people with whom she could talk equally. The intellectual people she did find did not match her spiritual dimension.

It is not wrong to be aware of our abilities in life. Awareness is a good thing. However, we should never be arrogant about our accomplishments. They are opportunities the universe has provided for us to improve ourselves and the world around us. They are merely tools.

If this woman is to find the friends that she desires, she needs to examine where they will be and get herself there. Where would she hang out? Also, she needs to be very clear on who she wants as a friend. What characteristics is she looking for? She should make a list and be very clear about what she really wants in order to get it. It is the law of the universe.

We don't get what we want when we are unclear. Whatever it is that you seek, make your list and read it to yourself every morning. Make a reality for yourself. The universe's timeline may be different from yours. Everything comes to you when it is supposed to, provided you don't put up roadblocks to prevent it from happening.

Patience is the paramount key to happiness. We need to understand the concept of our need for having everything right now versus having it when it is the right time. It is time for us to learn how to relax. I encourage you to find a qualified instructor to show you how to relax through breathing, stretching, and deep relaxation therapy. Practice it every morning and be honest with yourself. Why do you want something? Be clear.

# Fuel for the
# Body, Mind, Spirit

If we were centered in ourselves, then we could draw on that energy to establish relationships with others and still have plenty more to establish our own sense of worth. You can say to yourself, "I am going to sit down and write down a description of me." This is not a résumé. This would be a narrative description of you. It could be in the form of poetry. It could be a collage. It could be a personal essay. It is important to do this exercise to know where you are coming from. None of the descriptions should be about your relationship to someone else. For example, "I am a sister" is not what you are looking for. Instead look for descriptions of you independent of your relationships. This is where we usually end our self-description. But it is important to think of you, independent of everyone and everything else. Trying to do this exercise is just as instructional as actually completing your self-description. It will open yourself to questions and expand your vision of your capabilities.

This is how you fuel your body, mind, and spirit. You need to reclaim the energy that you use to serve the world around you. Instead, that energy could fuel you to be the person that best serves *your* needs. It if makes you feel better to do something for someone, then it is in your best interests to go ahead and do that; however, be clear in your mind about why you are doing it and how your energy is being used. Do not look for acknowledgment from the outside. Never do something because someone will react in a certain way. It may or may not happen. It is better to depend on yourself for gratification.

What fuels you? What do you take in with your five senses that makes you *you*? What would you need to see every day to feel great? What do you need to read? What do you need to hear? What do you need to taste? What do you need to feel? For example, feeling your mother's cheek on yours is a great feeling. It leaves you feeling more secure. You may need to read a certain article in the paper every day that leaves you with a smile on your face. Have you ever tried reading for therapy? Try changing how you feel by reading different things than what you are used to reading. A great cure for depression is to walk to the library and pick up any book and just start reading. Read something that you don't normally read consistently for fifteen minutes, and don't stop until fifteen minutes have passed. This is a positive strategy to feel better or at least different after this exercise.

We can easily change our moods by changing our thoughts; however, sometimes we are so addicted to the pity party that we let ourselves feel badly for longer than is necessary. Consider this analogy: You allow yourself the one chocolate in order to feel better. Then the emotional part of you realizes that if you continue to feel bad, you could have another chocolate. Hmmm. Sounds like a plan.

What we really need to do is to have something kick-start our brains and jettison the emotional baggage. This will fuel our day and make us more productive. One way of doing this is to watch something uplifting. Keep inspirational, motivational, or otherwise positive material on hand for such an occasion; however, make sure you don't spend hours watching YouTube and not thinking for yourself. Watch about an hour of something that is useful. We all have movies that make us feel better. Have four or five of these on hand. Choose from one of them and force yourself to get out of the emotional rut you are in. Don't dwell in it. No matter what your ego tells you, it is not a productive place to be. You need to realize this first and foremost. After watching an hour of your uplifting selection, take a pad and paper and write down what you liked about it. Write at least three points. Also try and write a paragraph about how you felt. Write at least ten lines, and force yourself to sit there in your place until you have finished writing them. There will be great resistance from within you because your internal self realizes the great potential of this exercise to make you so strong and powerful that it is unbelievable. But your smaller self would rather wallow and not allow your larger self to feel good. Watch out for this!

Have you ever read a book that was so interesting that for the time you were reading, you forgot the world? Or did you ever have a conversation with a friend and found that the time just rolled by and you'd hardly got started talking? These are instances that prove that moods can be changed by how your mind is operating. Let's use this concept. If we are feeling bad or depressed, we know this can be changed. We operate at three levels. They are body, mind, and spirit. Let's access our mood at one of these levels.

The fastest way to change your mood is to go for a long walk. It needs to be a half hour to an hour long in order to make changes in your mood. The longer the walk is, the more stable your mood changes are. You can think about anything during this walk. But there is something about being in touch with the elements that always changes your life, no matter what. It is like being in touch with nature and having it empathize with your problems. It is like talking to a silent observer. There is nothing like walking during a winter morning when everything is quiet. Even if it is thirty-five degrees outside, it is certainly invigorating and problem solving in nature. Ultimately you begin to discover what is really bothering you. This unravelling, in itself, is a major discovery.

# YOGA AS A TOOL FOR UPLIFTMENT

Yoga has been touted as being the answer to body-mind issues. But what exactly is it? What do people do in yoga that makes this the wonder drug? The word *yoga* is a Sanskrit word meaning "joined." What are we joining? That would imply that something is separate and needs to be joined. Usually we are a mass of body, and our mind is thinking a million other things, perhaps totally unrelated to our task at hand. Our spirit, or inspiration, is probably trying to communicate with us but can only do so when we are "tuned" to it or listening to it—existing not in the "do" world but in the "be" world. Being is important. Be yourself and in the moment, not reaching out to yesterday or tomorrow. The physical moves, or asanas, in yoga are the vehicle for that focus. When we breathe a certain way, we become more focused. These rules of breathing are dictated by the yoga science. It is a scientific work of documented methodologies of achieving this "unification" of body, mind, and spirit. Several books comprise the body of knowledge known as yoga science. These are Hatha Yoga Pradipika, Shiva Samhita, and Gherunda Samhita. The asanas are determined by a person's level in yoga. It is not about how your body can be contorted but how deep your breathing is and how focused you are while doing the asana. The length of time in a posture is determined by your level. Beginner participants should try for twenty seconds of focus. Intermediate participants should try for thirty seconds, and advanced participants can go beyond thirty seconds to their comfort zone for the moment. A person's level will change with time of day, mental makeup, and circumstances, perhaps the weather. So yoga is very much about being in touch with what you need that day, at that time.

This also tells us that everyone can do yoga by adjusting to his or her comfort level. Some people can use whatever aids they will need. I have conducted a yoga class with people sitting on chairs. Wrists are an issue for many people, so there are modifications for sore wrists as well. The instructor can modify asanas on the fly for the comfort and benefit of the participant.

Yoga makes changes in the body, mind, and spirit. We can affect our emotional moods through yoga. In fact, certain *yogasanas*, or postures, directly affect dyspepsia. This can be used in our favor.

# YOGA AS A CURE FOR DEPRESSION

We are usually feeling sorry for ourselves and that is why we feel depressed. It is a fear that we are alone and no one is out there to help us. Instead, we really need to turn this thinking around: *I am an able-bodied being with many gifts. What can I do to help the world around me?* More than likely, something will come up to help you establish your faith in yourself. It is like the boomerang effect. We feel love when we give it. We get presents when we give them. We are entertained when we entertain. We get opportunities if we give them. So next time you feel like you are not getting your share of something, try an exercise to see if you can give that. Attention is something we all crave, and we feel neglected when we don't get it. The next time that feeling comes, you might try to give attention to someone deserving. Surely there must be someone in your life who you feel deserves some attention for doing something nice or for just being an all-around nice person. Why not give that person a call? Arrange to take him or her out for coffee or lunch. Or simply just talk on the phone and tell him/her what a nice job you think he/she is doing.

Awards are funny. We go through life thinking we need some kind of recognition from the outside world. As long as that feeling exists, it is a sure thing that we feel like we are not completely serving the world at our maximum capacity. So increase the way in which you do whatever it is you do. If it is business attention you crave, then try to give it to someone who deserves it. Recognize yourself for what a great job you did this year. List all the things your company has done and pat yourself on the back. Take yourself out to lunch. Remember that you are your best company.

# FUEL YOUR BODY

Remember that you need fuel at all three levels. At the physical level, we know about physical fitness training. Of course, most people put the cart before the horse and dive into a gym with a fitness membership and sign their life away with a personal trainer. Instead, look at your eating and fix that first. Your money will be better spent if instead of giving it to your fitness trainer, you give it to someone who can seriously fix your eating habits to make a real difference in your life! Also, invest in a stress-reduction program. Take the cortisol levels down in your body so that you have a fighting chance against building up fat reserves. If you do these two things first, before the physical training program, you will set up the foundation so that your physical program can make a difference. Most people do this in reverse order or don't fix their eating and stress at all. This is why most people fail at "getting in shape."

To address physical fitness, you have to be smart about it. Don't waste time on a treadmill or other cardio device at a steady state and expect to burn off the pounds. Not going to happen. This is where you need an intelligent trainer to assess what *you* need—not a cookie-cutter program, but what *your* body needs. How is it going to get to the next level of fitness? Where is it now? A lot of people waste time chasing their idea of which fitness program would be good for them. The truth is there is no "one size fits all" in fitness, and really, you could be wasting a lot of time and get disappointed quickly if the time you've invested in training doesn't pay off. Invest in someone who can give you good advice. It is so worth it.

We can look at a few trends in training. Kettlebell training has become popular. A kettlebell is made of cast iron and consists of a ball with a handle attached to it. It is a unique Russian training system. The weights start at 8kg and usually go up in increments of 4kg. It is an exercise that uses lower body strength to propel your upper body to get stronger, but it has a steep learning curve. There is a risk of injury from bad form and bad instruction, hence the need for proper training with a good instructor. Kettlebell training aficionados claim to get fast results; however, we must first analyze their fitness ability. Perhaps a few months of endurance training and standard weight training protocol would warm up and prep the muscles for the demands of a kettlebell workout. Then you can really reap the benefits of the exercise. Again, you would have to get this information from a qualified fitness professional who can answer that question in person, by assessing your current fitness level.

Another great fitness trend is TRX. TRX is Total Resistance Exercise training. It is made of two straps that suspend from the ceiling or over a doorframe. It is mainly body weight training. In this case also, you may need to spend a few weeks building up your core strength and endurance. There is nothing wrong with spending time to get to a point where a training tool can make a difference. But if you are not scientific about your training, it will result in injury and make you depressed about your lack of progress in fitness as well.

Running is a great sport. Great-looking people like Jon Bon Jovi say they run six miles a day or have taken up yoga. There is no denying that some people have excellent genetics on their side. You have to take that into account. If your knees are not up to doing those miles, then taking up an activity because someone else has and looks great would be a recipe for injury. The message in all this is to do what is right for your body-mind-spirit combination. Again, you would need a professional to tell you this. It is worth getting an educated, objective opinion.

Weight training is great. But you need to know how fast to progress and what protocol in weight training progression is good for you. How much time do you have to train, and what are the results you want? These questions need to be answered to get to your goal in a practical amount of time without getting injured. Unfortunately, advertising being what it is, there are unreasonable-looking sports models being paid to advertise the latest training program. That doesn't mean that model got to looking like that using that program. It just means they are getting paid to advertise that program. In fact, they may not even use that program at all. A fitness professional would be able to tell you that information.

We need to have our body work at its optimum level. An optimum fitness level gives us the tools with which to carry out our day. It is the one tool we have at our disposal to manipulate. We seem to make time for eating and sleeping but never for physical fitness training. We take it for granted until the dreaded visit to the doctor at which time she tells you that you need to hire a trainer. It is a funny thing that the more we exercise, the more we crave it. I have clients who swear by their Sunday morning run. For them and for me, it is quiet "me" time. I can think through all the matters of the week. I can prepare for my week. It is exciting. It is truly a lovely time. If you have ever run on a cool winter morning when no one is yet up for their Sunday shopping, it is the most awesome experience. You meet the other runners who come out for that same experience. You have bonded with humanity and you think you can lift the world. After returning from this experience, you shower and feel like this was a day well spent already. If you do nothing else right today, you have at least invested some time in giving your body, mind, and spirit a treat. Way to go!

# FUEL YOUR MIND

Fuel for our mind is the next stop. By focusing only on our physical bodies, we ignore our minds' need for fuel. It is true that a lot of people have written about "brain smart" foods. That is only a small part of the total healthy mind picture. Eating a lot just makes you full and sleepy and may not answer the fundamental problem of efficient mental capability. Nutrition is a very important and confusing topic. Studying the various nutrition protocols out there can make us dizzy. One book says one thing is good, and the next expert says it is not. What are you going to eat?

Practicality is key here. First of all, you must get to a proper nutritionist that has a practical approach to eating and not fad-type food. There are a lot of foods that are good for you. For example, hemp seeds and chia seeds are undoubtedly good. However, can you do just as well from a proper eating plan? Can you stay away from fried food for six days of the week? Can you stick to your healthy eating plan 80 percent of the time? Then really that is all it takes. We all know to eat properly; we just don't do it. Instead, what you need to do is to promise yourself that one heavy carb day when you can eat nachos or whatever your food craving is. Then you know that is coming and will be motivated to eat properly the other days of the week.

The quantity you should eat is such that you will be mildly hungry in two to three hours. Have real food for lunch, for example, about a palm's worth of lean protein like Greek yogurt (approximately half a cup) and a couple of fistfuls of cooked fresh vegetables. Make sure the veggies are from home so they're fresh and don't have bloating preservatives. Your last meal should not be later than two hours before you go to bed. If you go to bed at 10:00 p.m., don't eat after 8:00 p.m. If you are hungry, opt for herbal tea. In these two hours, your desire for food is usually more of a comfort thing. All that eating food at this time of day will do is to make sure it sits undigested in your stomach. Try to eliminate sugar and processed carbohydrates, especially those items bought from fast-food outlets. Remember, sugar and chocolate cravings are comfort cravings. Do ten burpees or whatever it takes to get the endorphins up to combat the cravings. Do the water or herbal tea thing. Just get over it. You can do it. You have to exercise some willpower here.

# GETTING MENTAL ALERTNESS

We need to invest time in making our minds sharp. There are many tools to achieve this gradually. Like any physical exercise program, however, progress must be gradual. We must be patient with ourselves. Breathing exercises through yoga have the benefit of helping us to become calmer and more tolerant of the situations around us. Many clients have told me that they are much calmer in public after a few weeks of yoga involving breathing training. Our mental training program must entail reading, writing, and stretching.

Reading elevates the mind. If the material is enlightening, then the mental neural network gets active. We may find ourselves discovering the solution to a problem that we really have stopped thinking about. When we activate our mental world, then whatever other activities are happening in that space are accelerated as well. We must read a lot and read a variety of books often. One colleague told me she had always only read high-tech books for her job and because of her own interest in the area. She had always looked down upon fiction as something that was not realistic and therefore not worth reading. At some point, she took the plunge and started reading fiction for fun. She soon started seeing the world in a well-adjusted way. She lost the attitude of "my way or the highway" and became more tolerant of other people's views. She discovered the value of fiction.

Let us discuss this phenomenon: while fiction is truly not real, as the label implies, our brain can't tell the difference. Instead we read something first and then use a filter to determine whether we want to believe it or not. Then we decide where we are going to store it. It can go in the junk file, to be flushed. Otherwise, we put it in a file to be retained so we can think about it and refer to it later. What happens when we start getting interested in a story is that, even if our intellectual segment tells us it is junk, we may retain some of the sentiment obtained from reading what we enjoyed so we can recall the feeling at a later date. That gives us permission to dream. We need to dream. Without dreaming, there is no ingenuity. None of the discoveries we take for granted would be here if someone didn't dream. None of the products of the entertainment industry would be here if their creators didn't dream. We must be careful to entertain a variety of thoughts. If we always read the same type of book, it would be like eating only one type of donut all the time. We would be limiting our experience, and our mental space would get stale, having not obtained the correct stimulus for creativity.

# FUEL YOUR SPIRIT

Our spiritual side must be addressed for total body, mind, and spirit fitness to occur. Spirituality does not mean sitting in lotus position. It means being in touch with our real selves. Spirituality is not something that can be defined; however, we all know people who are "spiritual." They are somehow together. This means they know what their inner being is about. They will not lead you astray as to who they are. They usually beam confidence, and you can feel it. Their handshakes are strong. They are usually focused and get things done. They know where they are and where they need to go. Perhaps they are unsure about how to go about it but usually not for long. They will seek out those who can help them get there. It's all about knowing. It's all about being. I firmly believe that practice of writing in the morning will help you to become one of these people. You will be mentally well adjusted.

Breathing exercises in yoga teach us to become more integrated. We are not integrated when our breathing is erratic, shallow, and short. When we are relaxed, we find our breathing is regular, deep, and long. It is most efficient in this state. If you have ever watched a baby sleep, then you have observed the abdomen of the baby rising and falling deeply. Even watching a baby sleep is very calming for that reason. It is rhythmical and integrated breathing. Yoga develops our character integration. Clients have repeatedly told me how they have become more tolerant of the world around them after a few weeks of a proper yoga class.

We must keep in mind that the quality of yoga instruction is of paramount importance. It is important to be clear about the quality of instruction that you are receiving. Many people have complained of injuries after a yoga class. That is due to improper instruction alone. It is not possible to get injured with proper yoga instruction. Yoga instructors must undergo a rigorous amount of training in order to address the benefits and limitations of each asana or posture. For each asana there is a limiting population. You should also be aware of the benefits of each asana. They are not just designed to make you feel like you are doing yoga. In fact, the names of most postures have incorrect translations into English. Yoga was developed five thousand years ago in India, and the language used was Sanskrit. Sanskrit is still used today and the original language has power and should be retained. The inverted V posture, for example, with both hands and feet on the floor with the tailbone up in the air pointed toward the ceiling is frequently called "downward dog." However, it was at one point called Parvatasana, or mountain, where the thinking is that we look like a mountain and have uplifting thoughts while thinking of scaling a mountain or looking as tall as a mountain. A mountain is lofty and high reaching. We can think of the snowcapped Himalayas, which are ever inspiring, while doing the posture, for example. This serves to elevate the mind. Yoga is meant to cause spiritual evolution. Spiritual evolution yields the byproducts of mental and physical health.

# Wholesome Living

We must think of ourselves as human beings: *I am a human being. I am just hanging out here.* Our other relationships serve our purpose; each of these must be defined for ourselves in the context of how and to what extent.

I once knew a woman who complained about her friend Joe. Let's say the woman's name is Susan. She complained that Joe did not call her often. He would not communicate with her enough. Susan wondered what was wrong. She asked him to communicate with her, say, once a day; however, she would not hear from him. I asked her what this friendship was. Was it defined in some format? Was it more than friends? Were they both clear on what form the relationship was supposed to take? It is when things are in the fuzzy zone that we don't know where to put the relationship. Susan had to decide what she wanted this relationship to be and then act in that manner.

Clarity is essential for relationships to move forward. Otherwise they cause drama that doesn't need to be there. Of course, I know a lot of people that crave drama; however, it really is not a great use of energy. You can save that energy for other things that are more productive—perhaps becoming the next great novelist or next great community bar piano player. The choices are endless as to how you can use your energy. Eventually Susan chose to chuck Joe from her life altogether and move on. Their relationship was just another energy drain that she didn't need. It is not important what happens to Joe. If you think it is, then you just crave drama. You have to evaluate your needs. If the world doesn't serve you to accomplish those needs, and instead creates an energy deficit that is not worth it, then you need to reevaluate and move on. At the time of this writing, Joe is still confused but not creating any confusion in Susan's life. Of course, if Joe decides to seek coaching, then I would be happy to help him sort out what it is he is really after.

In our mind space, each of our relationships with others need to be filed; otherwise it hangs around causing havoc and interrupting our other activities, asking for a resolution or an answer to the question of what that relationship is supposed to be. It is unfinished and undefined. The mind hates stuff like that. It wants to neaten up everything and put it away somewhere.

When you are unclear about something, then things can torment you. You need to take time to sort it out and free up much-needed RAM (in computerspeak: Random Access Memory or free space) for important decisions. This is where the energy drain comes in. Energy that is needed for important things, like yourself, is relegated to figuring out why someone said something to you and what you felt about that. You need to spend time refueling yourself. You need this car to run so you need to fuel it each day in a proper way. Spend time on yourself. Figure out the proper amount of nourishment that's required for you to function properly throughout the day. Then give yourself permission to follow through on that "me schedule." You will thank you.

How much do you need to refuel? What amount is enough? Consider the whole you, which incorporates your body, mind, and spirit. Each part acts on one another. You need to consider each aspect so that the whole you will be happy and well balanced. You need physical exercise. This feeds into a mental and spiritual state. You need nutritional guidelines for your body type, disposition, and eating habits. There are professionals who design these guidelines and can recommend training programs for you. This is what a personal trainer does. Get the information that you need to make those informed decisions. You also need to address your mind. Are you feeling stressed out? How can you rearrange life so that you are more relaxed? Do you need to do it all, right now? What intellectual stimulation do you need and how much is necessary for your daily happiness? Be sure to build that into your lifestyle. There are people who stagnate because they never focused on their intellectual needs. Indeed, you also need to address your spiritual needs. Whatever you find motivating, inspirational, and beyond description is spiritual for you. It need not be organized religion. It is creativity and inspiration.

Speculating on why someone did something is a certain way to set yourself up for failure. Focus on you and resist the urge to speculate on someone else. Think of what you need. This might be a hard exercise for some. If you think, *I am never going to let him get away with this*, then you are just making yourself miserable. Forget about the other person. What do *you* want? Most people in relationships play this game and end up making both parties miserable. You need to drop the second-guessing of the other person's actions. This is what causes pain. It is also wasted energy. Instead, sit down and think, *What do I want?* Once you determine your answer, ask for what you want plainly.

We often think about our happiness in terms of what others can do for us. Instead, we need to think of how happy we would be from our own actions. If we make dinner for some guests, then we should not feel happiness from their appreciation of the event. Instead, we need to feel happiness from the act of entertaining itself. It is like they are not really there at all. They are like pictures on a canvas that we have painted. In a flash you can make them disappear. Characters outside of us are our impressions of them. Their real personality is most probably something entirely different from how we may perceive them. For example, someone who is not saying much isn't necessarily angry at you. They are probably preoccupied with some other issue. Preoccupation also sometimes comes across as being tired. Their face doesn't reflect the same amount of joy, perhaps. We read too much into other people's actions and thoughts and make ourselves miserable.

How do we focus on ourselves instead of constantly saying the outer world does not behave properly? We need to practice this skill. Every day, for a week, write out how something you did made you happy. The description must be all about your activity and your feeling. There should be no other parties' actions involved in this description. This exercise builds the ability to make yourself happy in all situations. When you are depressed, it is entirely up to you to get yourself out of it. We convince ourselves that it is our boss or colleague, for example, who is making us unhappy. In actuality, it is our perception of the event that causes us grief.

If you worked at making yourself happy every day and did the things that satisfy you, more than likely that you will be happy. Happiness is never an outside force. It is an internal force. We often read in the news about millionaires who are depressed. We often think that if we had the amount of money that they possessed, then everything would be perfect and we would be happy all the time. However, many of them are depressed and have social issues. If it is not one lack, it is another lack that we identify, and this constant focus on what we don't have is what makes ourselves depressed.

Wholesome living is a way to live with the proper attitude. It is a way of life. We need to assess each part of our life and take action. If money is lacking, then we must devise a plan and act it out. Taking action is a great way to fend off depression or unhappiness. Wallowing in negative emotions is a surefire way of staying depressed. Fear is a great force, and we need to get rid of it any which way we can.

One way of getting rid of fear is by writing. If we constantly write down how things should be, what we write will eventually happen because the mind is very powerful. Anything we think does happen. However, when what we desire is something good, we hamper it by thinking of the opposite in a more powerful way. For example, we may think, "Wow, this is a great job opportunity. I am going to apply for it right now. But what if the competition is better?" Instead, we can write down what we think would be great for us. This technique overcomes the negative forces and has a chance of happening. By putting in place an offense that's powerful, it will drown out the negative talk that your mind will come up with. The question is when? That is determined by how strongly we will it to be. If we say to ourselves, "My house is straightened up and tidy, and I can actually find everything," then in the next breath we say, "Oh that could never be possible. I have too many more important things to do," we are actually creating a negative balance by decreasing the power of the positive thought about cleaning up. Of course, cleaning up is important. We need to be able find everything. More importantly, good energy comes from our living space being tidy. We need to focus on what makes the machine operate smoothly. We have a tendency, instead, to plug along, hoping to get through the day. Obviously, we can do better than that.

# REAL MEANING OF WHOLESOME LIVING

Wholesome living is living intentionally. It is not hoping that five o'clock comes around so you can go home and lie on the couch. Then you are just waiting for bed and dreading getting up the next morning. Is this any way to live? Think of your talents. The world is indeed missing out because of your pathetic attitude. If you feel you have nothing to offer, then challenge yourself. For five minutes, write down everything that is good about you. Then read it over to yourself every morning. Even on days when you don't feel like it, read it over to yourself anyway.

Another thing that is quite surprising is the number of people who do nothing about taking care of their physical body. Are they hoping it will take care of itself? Can you imagine driving your car every day for a year and hoping it will run? Can you imagine fueling it with the contents of your garbage and hoping it will run? I am sure that everyone will answer in the negative to these questions. Even the most miserly of us will take the car in for an oil change. On days when the dirt is exceptionally bad, we take the car in and get it washed. Otherwise, we would not be able to see out the windows. We all have noticed people who we drive behind and wonder if they can see us because their rear window is covered in grime. It is a wonder.

However, people don't even take the time to consult an expert about their health and training for daily use. People should go to their doctors and have them assess their physical health. What is stopping people from seeking a professional fitness trainer for an assessment and recommendations for lifelong health? This is a question everyone needs to answer. We must learn to take care of the one thing that enables us to get through every second of every day. That is our body, and these bodies include our minds and spirits. Wholesome living is how we take care of ourselves so that we may take care of the world around us. Think of the CEO of a major corporation. How effective can he be if he has a physical ailment? Can he perform at his maximum capacity? Obviously the answer is no. He is limited by the extent to which he has cared for his body, mind, and spirit. These three components of a human being work together to generate our performance in the outside world. These three components don't work independently; that is why we cannot neglect one in favor of another.

How do you seek out a professional fitness trainer that is going to be beneficial to you? There are many trainers out there. The best way to find one is to ask around. Ask each person you know who has a trainer about his or her experiences. Does the trainer provide individualized instruction, or is it the same cookie-cutter program that he gave the last five clients? Does the trainer compensate for injuries? Is he linked in to other health-care professionals like chiropractors, physiotherapists, and massage therapists? Is he qualified to give out nutrition advice? How physically fit is the trainer? What does he do to keep up, and what professional credentials does he have? How does he improve on his knowledge base in the fast-growing fitness industry? Do his peers acknowledge his abilities? In other words, what do other trainers think of him? Take the time to find the trainer that is right for you.

A word of caution: most trainers who work in commercial (franchise) gyms usually are experiencing pressure to sell sessions. Be aware and think for yourself. You may want to get assessed by several trainers before making your decision about who will work best with you. If a trainer is about selling sessions, you will have to think hard about what you are getting. This may not be bad, but you need to be aware of quality before signing up for multiple sessions and then being disappointed.

There are people who live at the gym. What are they accomplishing? It might as well be a pub that they are sitting at. They fool themselves into thinking that this is time well put in. However, I wonder if they see any difference in their physical fitness level. I have seen people do the same exercises day after day, with no progress in weights or physical ability. It doesn't look to me like their workouts are accomplishing anything. The first step is to see an expert and get an analysis of the program tailored for the individual. Some types of exercise do nothing for some people. Their conditioning prevents them from seeing results at that level. If they were to take their exercise up a notch, they would definitely see results.

Have you ever wondered why some people rave about certain gyms that have circuit training based on pace exercise? Their physiology responds to that. For some people, that is like a walk in the park. For others, it may be the first time they have ever worked their body and they will come out of that workout with a deep sense of having accomplished something. Be critical about your trainer and your training. Compare. Ask questions. Why are you doing something? Know that there is no "one size fits all" in fitness training. There is no one diet that will solve everyone's nutritional issues. There is no one spiritual training that will enable everyone to grow. You need to seek out people who will help you get there, and everything they instruct you to do has to be individualized for *you*.

# Many Problems, One Solution

We need to realize that the whole being is interconnected. The body affects the mind, which affects the spiritual being. Similarly, the subtler levels of our being affect the mind and body. We cannot work in isolation. We cannot address a problem with only one aspect of our being.

For example, many people want to become more fit, and in that process, they think of losing weight. It is interesting that many people identify fitness levels with losing weight. What is more important is individual health. If the individual's maximum heart rate is being jeopardized by their weight, then weight management would be a necessity in order to maintain health. Otherwise, weight should not be the first issue that is addressed. The more important question is: How healthy are you? That is something everyone should be interested in. Weight is not a good measurement of health. It should never be the barometer by which we determine good health. Why do we look at thin women and say to ourselves that they have nothing to worry about? In fact, thin people have to understand the necessity of strong bones. Limiting nutrition will not make sure your bones are strong.

Look at yourself from a health standpoint. Are you healthy? Could you be healthier? This means, is there a way to improve your health so that you are more alert and able to take on the activities of the day in an effective manner?

Write a description of your perfect day. What would you wear? What would you eat? Who would you talk to? Don't let practicality enter the story. Just ask yourself: What would I love to do? This opens up that part of you that is aching to get out. Try to understand what makes you happy. Face that as well. Don't make editorial comments about it. If watching old movies makes you happy and you can escape into another world with them, then accept that fact. Own it. Declare it proudly. It is who you are. It is wonderful. The thing to note is that which makes us feel great appeals to all of our senses. We are integrated beings when we feel something connect with us. It is not possible to describe it in words. You are just feeling from within. Make it yours and own it.

Our problems really do boil down to that one phenomenon of integrating the body, mind, and spirit. We must become integrated in body, mind, and spirit. We need to find ways to feel well adjusted and interface with the outside world in a positive and productive way. We must engage ourselves in practices that develop our bodies, minds, and spirits.

Physically, we would all benefit from the services of a qualified professional fitness trainer. We need our trainers to critically assess where we are and where we need to go in order to stay healthy. If we are merely left to our own devices, then we may hurt ourselves. There is no one physical fitness program that suits everyone. It really must be tailored. You also want to streamline your efforts. You don't want to be wasting time. For example, beginners typically waste time in the weight room. People are looking for ways to tone their body. They pick up a book on weight training. The book is probably designed with an audience of those experienced in weight training in mind. Therefore, the book might prescribe doing many sets of a particular resistance-training exercise. Beginners would be prone to increased injury if they followed this advice. Their muscles are newly getting acquainted with the whole idea of training in general. The excitement of results leads them to overtrain and get injured. Instead, find a trainer that can show you the best way to effectively use your time to train for your physical condition.

Mentally, you need to understand what your mind is up to. If you do not carry out this type of introspective analysis for your mind, then you may lead a confused and nonintegrated life. You must strive to be well adjusted. The best way to achieve this mental integration is through writing therapy. In *The Right to Write*, author Julia Cameron has a great recipe for writing when she advocates the Three Morning Pages, as we discussed earlier. This system tells people that they should write three pages in the morning. This is not writing for others to see. Instead, it is an outpouring of your mind's contents. On the page you answer the question, "What are you thinking about?" Just write and don't edit your writing. Nothing is too bad or too good to write. It simply is. At this time, you get to understand what your mind is worried about. Write it down even if it seems nonsensical. There is no room for editorial comment here. If you had an argument or disagreement with someone, write it down. Try to understand yourself. That is the goal of writing. It is you getting in touch with you.

Recently a climber to Everest told me he had trouble with his last climb. His problem was not physical. Instead, he was not prepared mentally for the trip. This time around, he wanted the tools to be there within himself and he wanted to experience the moment in a better way. When most people think about climbing Mount Everest, they think of the physical challenges involved. Indeed, the physical challenges are not to be ignored in order to survive the journey and the return trip. And while it is true that a climbing expedition is a group effort, each person has to be with him or herself during the trek. You can't climb and carry on a conversation with your buddy as you would during a Sunday morning run in the park. First, there is the physical distance between you and the next person on the rope that supports the unity of the team. Second, climbing is an individual effort. It is demanding. It requires preservation of oxygen. It is like being the frontline marathoner in a race. You need to conserve your energy to make it. In the background of your mind is the return trip, and conservation is a critical factor for survival. Mental toughness is not enough. There in the vast expanse of cold and snow, you meet yourself. It better not be for the first time. Otherwise your mind will not permit you to go farther. At the time when you are with yourself, you need to train your mind to be comfortable with its own company. This is yoga.

An integrated person can deal with any situation. There are no boundaries. Life is life. There is no delineation between work and home. Often you see the phrase "work/life balance" being used. It seems to say that work is not life. It is. Life is everything we do in the twenty-four hours of every day we are alive. Even sleeping is life. How we sleep represents who we are. If we are sound sleepers, then it shows that we have managed to integrate our personality. We choose not to worry about those things that bother us. However, if we don't sleep well at night, then it shows that we are carrying our worries with us. We have not processed all the information that is in our brain. Yoga and breathing is the answer here. We must learn to breathe properly. Breathing helps align our body. We function in a more integrated fashion if we learn to breathe. Normally we hide our stress in various areas of our body. Breathing helps relieve that stress and prevents it from building up.

The client who was climbing Mount Everest told me his arms and shoulders were tight from lifting weights. It was not from stress; therefore, to him it was okay. It was going to help him climb. But tightness is tightness. It does not help us in any way. Lifting weights does build strong and hard muscle and takes out the flabbiness. It is strength that we need when climbing. However, I wondered about the rishis who live in the Himalayas. They do yoga for hours at a time. They are strong. They can withstand the elements. They hardly wear any clothing while living in a very cold climate. I walk outside when it is -35°C and my nose feels like it is going to fall off. I can barely feel my fingers. From yoga I know that this is just a state of mind. Pain and pleasure are in the mind. That is how the yogis can do meditation in cold climates that are unbearable for human skin. You can put your mind somewhere else and enable your body to weather anything. Therefore, there is a great lesson for us. If something *seems* like pleasure, it is just that. It seems like pleasure. If something *seems* painful, it is just that. It is not really painful. It just seems painful. To someone else with a different perspective, it is pleasure.

This Mount Everest story tells us of the great role the mind plays in life. It is the maker or breaker. Ever notice how you are interested in a TV show, yet your mind wanders? Then you wonder what happened to the half hour as the credits roll for the show. It truly is incredible. I once had a cosmetologist who had to give a local anesthetic to my face. Facial muscles are not tough, and that kind of needle hurts immensely. I trained myself to take my mind away from the pain. I actually dove into the pain and accepted it. It minimized the pain immensely. But I was in meditation. The doctor was wondering what happened to me. Did I pass out? He was not aware of the power of meditation. He got scared that he had lost a patient and kept prompting me to "say something." However, I once had a dentist who gave me an anesthetic in my mouth and, seeing me not react to it, concluded that it was because of "years of meditation." He did understand that I was aware of everything but chose to dive into meditation. The mind is a powerful tool. It really can make heaven of hell and hell of heaven. Believe it and learn how to use it.

When I was going through school, I would meet up with adults who would wistfully think back to how great school days were. From their perspective, school days were more carefree than their current situation in which they are responsible for their households. Perspective is everything. I was listening to them and thought to myself, *they don't remember how hard teachers are.* But really, they did remember. Only in comparison was that life better than the responsibilities of today.

We think we have many problems, but we have one problem: it is the mind. If we can control the mind through meditation, then we can conquer anything. If it is a physical issue such as weight gain, then we know if we think ourselves through what is causing the weight gain, we can get a handle on it. We need to find out what is causing the physical issue. Usually it is a response to an issue that is taking up our mental space. Instead of dealing with it at the mental level, we feel that eating will take our mind away from it. This is temporary. Now, not only have we not solved our mental problem, but we have added to it by creating a physical problem on top.

# The Big Secret

If you slow down and center your energy in you, then your relationships will develop in a more beneficial way to you. This is the secret. You could solve all your relationship problems on a case-by-case basis. Or you could center your thinking in you. This is energy well invested. Your relationships will take a different turn if you start looking at things from a you-centered approach. If you take the approach of "He makes me sooooo mad," then your attention will be on changing his character. Your positive mood is then dependent on when his actions are in line with your thinking. When is this going to happen?

Let's start by analyzing the statement "He makes me sooooo mad." Now, if "he" makes me mad, then "he" can make me happy. So if he says to you, "Happy. Be happy. Be happy" and waves his hands in front of your face, are you then happy? It will only happen if you let yourself want to be happy. Give yourself permission to be happy all the time. It has nothing to do with him. It was you all the time. You want to be happy, and so you are happy. You want to be angry, so you find something that makes you angry.

In order to step out of this outer world deciding what your inner world should feel, you need to step out of that circle of attention. Put more attention on yourself. What do you want? What do you need right now to make yourself happy? The outer world is there to help you get what you need and want. It serves you in the way you want it to. By emotionally lashing out at the outer world or some element of it, you are not solving the real problem. The real problem lies within you. You are actually angry at yourself: *Why can't I be* [insert phrase here]?

Now let's examine the old idea "Why can't I be like her?" Where is this thinking going to get you? First, what is lacking in you that makes you feel a need to be like someone else? Sit down and write down as many pages as you can on why you need to be like "her." Somewhere in there lies the secret of your success. Suppose it is because she seems to be self-composed and well-adjusted in all circumstances. You never see her mad. She seems to make courageous decisions about her life, which you wish you could emulate.

Okay, so now we are getting somewhere constructive. Instead of wasting your energy on finding a way to get back at her and grind your teeth, you need to find out how to develop those characteristics. Your other option is to simply accept the fact that we all have characteristics others admire and we all have personality traits we dislike about ourselves and want to change. So we can admire those traits in others and feel confident about our own set of positives within us. This admiration actually will cause us to slowly imbibe those traits. This is a very positive approach.

However, if you truly want to be as composed and calm as someone else, you need to be comfortable with yourself. If not, you are nervous in many situations. The best way to be composed and well-adjusted is to develop a sense of confidence in your own strengths. The best way to do this is to write. Write until the cows come home. Make this writing as detailed as possible. You can say, for example, "I once said to a friend who looked a little down, 'Hey, what's wrong?'" This would qualify as a demonstration of positive traits (caring, empathy). Be proud of your good qualities. They will carry you through life. This is the secret.

# HOW TO BRING OUT THE BEST IN YOU

Bringing out the best in you is the big secret. Our little self wants to squash anything good. It wants us to feel like there is no way and no escape. Instead we have to bring out the strength within us to conquer that lower self and rise above it. Have you ever had a friend who was petty and so you hated being around her? Did you avoid her like the plague? We have an inner petty person inside us. That person exists within us. She comes up to squash our great ideas. If we grow and become prosperous, we will surprise ourselves. That might be scary. I once met someone who suddenly made a lot of money. It surprised him and caught him off guard. He got nervous and gave it away. The presence of all that money presented his self with incredible possibilities. He could invest it and live off the interest for the rest of his life. *Wait a minute. Not having to go to work? No more being tied down to my job? But that is all I know.* That individual never developed a relationship with money. This sounds intriguing. A good example would be a musician and his or her instrument. Have you ever heard a musician talking about her instrument as if it were a living companion? The musician has established a relationship with the instrument. Similarly, if you want something to serve you well, then you must develop a relationship with it. Money is no exception. If you want money, then develop a relationship with money.

First, identify what your current relationship with money is. Then assess it to determine if you need to spend some time on that aspect of your life. This is a great opportunity to understand your ideas about money. A great exercise for this is to do the following. Take a plain sheet of paper. Write down what you would do if you suddenly received $100,000. How would your life change? Write the things down unedited. Don't critique your choices. You don't *have* to do anything in life. This is you and your paper talking to each other. No one else is going to see this. It is a discovery zone for yourself. Then do the same exercise with $50,000. Repeat the exercise with $25,000. Stop when you think the amount is actually something that you can handle. Stop the exercise when the amount doesn't seem outrageous. For some this could be $1,000. For others they might feel they need to go down to $25. It is irrelevant what the amount is. Keep this information for future reference. This is your relationship factor with your money. It reveals a lot about you. You may feel that a part of your personality is stunted because money was the thing you were waiting for. In actual fact, that is just the ego's way of stopping you from realizing your full potential.

Be practical about money. Talk to an expert. Find a good one by talking to people who are satisfied with their money strategist. Make a plan. Get out of any negative situations that you are in by talking to professionals who can help you make a plan. This is important for peace of mind. It all plays into fitness. Seriously, this is the one area where people think they are fine, only to discover that their Achilles' heel and stressor is in this one topic. How do you view those with money?

Fear is a big factor in our lives. We rationalize our lives around fear. I know people who are afraid to close their eyes. They have never met themselves. Meet yourself. It is a good idea to know who you are and where you stand before you thrust yourself on the outside world. After you meet yourself, you get a better idea of who you would be compatible with and who would bring out the worst in you. I once had a supervisor who brought out all the things in me that were negative for me. It took me some time to recognize that there are just going to be such people around and I can't do anything about them. I can, however, remove myself from their environment.

Attract what encourages and uplifts you. If you feel you are always surrounded by negative people, then the problem is you and not them. Realize this as your first step toward evolution. If you want to grow and be the person you can be, then you must attract toward you that which will create a good environment for you to grow. Do this exercise every day: just write down that you deserve encouraging people around you. Write down that you deserve a positive atmosphere around you. Keep doing this until you can change the forces around you. Be unswerving when it comes to what positive things you deserve. Don't ever settle. There is no such thing. It is simply making yourself the martyr, and there is no reason to waste a perfectly good person on that kind of a life. Say to yourself that you deserve the best that life can give. You attract around you what you think. So if you are surrounded by elements that you consider negative, then it is your own fault.

The big secret is basically that your world reflects what you think it is. If you are low in business, then you must change your thinking. It means that you think no one wants or is ready for your business. This thinking can be changed to say that everyone wants your business. It is only a matter of time before clients come to you. Figure out who or what your perfect client is. Then say to yourself that those clients are coming to you now. Understand that it is only your thinking that is stopping you from success. Success is yours. Just think that, and it will be true. Even now, send your energy to your perfect clients, and they will literally ring your phone and flood your inbox. Watch. It really is so.

You can help this process along. Don't sit alone in your house and complain that there are no clients. Get out and network. But target your networking. Don't go to an event where the attendees don't meet your client profile. That would be a waste of time and frustrating for you. Instead, go to events where you think there is a chance that your clients will be there. Then just be yourself. Don't sell. Just be there. Be open and don't panic at these events. Say to yourself, "I am here and am giving these people the opportunity to get to know me. I am going to get to know some nice people." There it ends. If there is a business connection, then it will happen. Forcing something is bad for everyone. Just be there and be present. Keep your mind focused on getting to know people in the room. If you make a connection, then that is great. If not, then you realize that now is not the time for them. However, they did get to know you. That is better than sitting at home, when those people didn't know you.

What are you complaining about? What do you feel is lacking in your life? Sit down and design how life would be with that element in it. Be descriptive of that person or thing that you feel would make your life better. Read this description over to yourself every morning. Let it sink in. Then watch it happen. A lot of women I know complain that they don't have the right man in their life. The solution is to be more precise. What do you mean by "right man"? Do you really mean that you would like a handyman that you don't have to hire? If so, then be honest with yourself. Write down what that person would look like and what characteristics he needs to have to make you happy. Read this over to yourself, as well, and remind yourself of the description of the person every morning. Then be open to that kind of person entering your life. It works. But you do have to leave the timeline to the universe. That is when you have to let go of the process. Just be grateful when it does arrive.

People complain about their jobs but they don't really know what they want. The big secret is simply to write down what you want. The big secret is fearlessness. We usually don't get what we want because we are afraid to get it. I was building a website a while ago. I knew that the website would be famous and produce many leads. I hesitated to do the write up for the sections for a long time. Fear of success crippled me. But I needed to face that fear. I wrote down that I knew it was because of fear of success that I didn't make progress on the writing. I told myself to just write every day. So it got finished. We all need to face our fears in order to make progress and open the door to our success.

# What Makes You Happy?

You need to understand what makes you happy. Have you ever had a case where something outside yourself made you happy, only to find it was temporary? The next moment, you find you are thrown into depression. It is at moments like this that you wonder about long-lasting happiness.

Pretend you were truly happy. Close your eyes and imagine yourself as being truly happy. What do you see yourself doing? What do you hear? What do you smell? Do you see yourself calm or excited?

True happiness is a state of mind. We liberate ourselves of all of our mental baggage. Our inner light shines. That's where true happiness comes from.

Most people cannot be happy because they harbor negative emotions. They are constantly looking for something or someone outside to make them happy. Of course, these events produce limited effects. No one person can make you happy all the time. In order to rid yourself of the negative emotions, there must be a lot of self-analysis. Your own internal conflicts prevent you from being happy. Therefore, you need to focus on how to ferret out your anger and resolve it. The best exercise for this is to close your eyes and repeat something that is uplifting. If you have a faith-based statement, you can repeat that. Otherwise, an inspiring statement like one of the following can be used:

a)  I am important to me.

b)  I am worth investing in.

c)  I am well adjusted.

d)  I interact with the world in a positive way.

e)  The future is positive.

f)  Good wishes are all around.

If you have never done this kind of practice before, then start with five minutes or even one minute.

This process of repetition should span a minimum of fifteen to twenty minutes. The most optimum amount of time is an hour. It would consist of four cycles of fifteen minutes interspersed with breathing. During the repetitions, your mind will wander. It is the nature of the mind to wander. However, it is important for you to note where it wanders to. These are the "hang-ups" that are holding you back. So the first part of identification is happening at this stage. It is important for you to be aware of your mind's contacts. They are what determine your level of happiness at any given time. Therefore, you need to understand what it is that is standing between you and your happiness. When thoughts interfere with your repetitions, you need to note what those are. You can mentally note them, or keep a pad and pencil near you at the time of meditation. Remain aware of what is going on with you. Your lack of awareness is what makes you angry at the wrong targets. This produces undesirable ramifications.

# HOW TO GET TO "HAPPY"

Why do we crave happiness? It makes us feel good. Can we generate that internally? That would make us happy all the time. We would no longer strive for things outside ourselves that make us happy. What a great way to be. Do you know people who already live like this? It is good to have role models when you think that this is not possible. It is possible. Truly dive deep and find that happiness within you. You will never go astray.

Our depression usually comes from feeling that the outside world should somehow cough up all the things that make us happy. When we don't get immediate gratification, we get depressed. However, depression is really another form of fear. We are afraid of what will happen if we don't get what we want. Our minds start spinning stories about the outcome, as if it would be disastrous for us. In order to get to our weakest point, the stories surround that. For example, if we are concerned about our finances, then our minds will convince us of a great story. We say, "If I don't get this job, then I won't have enough money to pay the rent." That is a pretty fearful consequence, and so the fear factor works against our clear thinking. How do we escape this spiral nose dive?

First, we need to calm down. It is very difficult to calm down in the face of such dire consequences. So we have to trick our minds. You may ask yourself, "Why do I want to calm down? I have to answer to these horrible consequences." Indeed you do. However, if you don't calm down, then even answers that are staring you in the face will not be obvious to you because your mind is wrapped up in the arms of the ego. This is a place where clear thinking will never come to be.

Writing is usually a good way to get out of fear or anger. We can vent on paper and get it out of our system. Usually it takes about three pages before we really find out what is going on with us. On the page, we can be honest. We can admit to ourselves that there are aspects to our being that we don't want to face.

When you do this exercise, be completely honest with yourself. If you don't like someone, then say so. Don't couch it in pretty language or justify it in any way. Don't say that person did something to you and therefore you are angry. Just say you don't like that person, and leave it at that. Write about happy things, too. Some people feel that they should not be happy. I once had a boss who never admitted that he was relaxing or enjoying an experience. He would always reword it to say he was in pain or suffering. Don't fool the world. There is no need. Just be honest with yourself. If you are happy about something, then it is okay to say that.

Happiness makes us feel good. Finding ways to make ourselves happy is what life is all about. We chase after many things from the time we wake up to the time we go to sleep; that is our modus operandi. We hardly take the time to analyze if that is what we really want or if it is just temporary relief. If we let ourselves do the analysis, then we would find the harsh reality that the activity that we are considering is really not going to get us what we need. It really is difficult to look past the pain and find out what we truly want. It is not a bad idea to seek the advice of a professional. The world is full of coaches ready to help us. We can inquire whether they will be able to talk to us to discover what is missing. This is not an exorbitant adventure. If you do your homework first as outlined in this book, then you will be ready to get that objective opinion from a professional.

It is truly amazing how people are willing to spend money on frivolities and then think it to be a waste of money to get their head straightened out. That is the wonder of life, of course. We really don't want to take the bull by the horns and get out of our misery. We would rather whine about it to anyone who listens. As long as we have an excuse, we don't have to do any real work.

# HOW TO TAKE THE BULL BY THE HORNS

Look at your life. It is a great book to read. Understand the experiences you've had. When I was doing graduate work, I thought it was hell on Earth. "Why am I not making progress?" I kept asking myself. I then realized that I was too focused on results. We all do this. We say to ourselves, "If this happens, then I will concentrate on my life." It is as if some magic needs to happen before we focus on developing ourselves. We always put the cart before the horse. Life experiences are for developing ourselves. If something is not coming forth, then we have to think that two things are happening: The first thought that we would entertain is that we are chasing after the wrong thing. The second thought is that we need to be more positive about the thing we are trying to do. We need to feel deserving of it so that it will come to us in its own time. Everything is ours for the asking. Only we don't ask correctly. We don't feel that we deserve it.

How do you undo the "wrong" thinking? By writing, by practicing yoga and meditation with a professional who can teach you the right way, by thinking positively, and by honestly seeing yourself as you are. Perhaps you are just not meant for what you seek at the time you seek it. Chuck your ego aside temporarily and really see the situation. Professionals are there to help you, and sometimes you have to spend some time and money to get the answers. Otherwise you risk wandering down a road that leads nowhere.

How do we feel that we deserve something so that we can make progress? We have to use the writing technique. If we write down that we deserve something, then we will begin to believe it. It is the first step. Our minds work in funny ways. If we see something in print, then we feel that it is true. More so, there is the power of our hand writing something down. It tends to make our nerves believe that we are engraving it in our mind space. What a great place to start. Believe it now. What are the alternatives? Feeling miserable is not an option.

Look at the ones whom you admire. Dream day and night. You can be great, too. By looking at the people you admire, you are more in touch with the greatness you aspire to exhibit. It is just a matter of pulling it out of yourself. Never feel that you can't do something. You can do everything. You just don't believe it right now. The goal of life is to believe. Crave happiness. When life gets you down and you feel weighted, do something else that day. When I was doing my doctorate work, I would go to the Ontario Science Centre and hang out. It was worth it. It took my mind off my problems. It turns out that I was worrying too much about results and battling the negative people who projected my own negativity. Remember that negative people are reflections of your own negativity.

The first thing that you should do when you feel negative is to seek out positive people and act positively around them. Temporarily suspend your negative ideas and bring out of yourself, by extrusion, the positive you. You can do this. Remember that mind is everything. It makes or breaks our life. There are myriad stories of hard-luck people making it big. Walt Disney was one of them. The original founder of the coffee retailer Second Cup was a drunk on the street. Now he is a millionaire and talks about his life. He also understands what it means to struggle. A great exercise to do at this stage is to sit down with yourself for fifteen minutes and write down all the things that are troubling you. Sometimes writing down your thoughts is therapeutic enough for you to see your way around what's blocking you.

Another trick is to think of one person who has what you crave. Then try to understand if you think that person is happy. What is it that they crave? I once thought that if I had more clients and more business, I would have it made. I would be happy. However, I immediately thought of someone who had two jobs and worked six days a week. This person's financial situation was never a concern; however, she was not happy. She craved time with family and downtime. I certainly had a satisfying amount of those items, and I really was happy. It really is our ego that makes us think we are unhappy. In reality, this is not the case. Refuse to believe this lie.

# BUILD AN IMAGE OF YOU

Who do you want to be? What is it that you find lacking in you right now, which prevents you from being in your image of success? Let's write that image down, but remember to phrase it positively—recording what you want to have rather than what you feel is lacking. Note the elements that make up that image. Are they things? Or is the list composed of statements of being? For example, did you write down that you are always cheerful? That could be a very good image of a successful person. Let's say you met someone at a party. What is it about that person that would define success for you?

Let's look at some examples. Suppose you met someone at a gathering who was angry at the world. This person was wealthy and had an excellent job and position in society. Everyone in society looked up to him. He was respected everywhere he went. However, he was bitter and angry. He grew tired of everyone's company. He didn't appreciate anyone. He had no friends, or at least no close friends. He didn't like his physical appearance. He gained a significant amount of weight and didn't take the steps to control that, although help was readily available. He had great spiritual ideas but never took the time to develop them. He would never be happy; true happiness was something he did not understand. He rushed everywhere and complained constantly about the lack of time.

Now suppose you met another individual at this same gathering. She had inordinate domestic problems. Her partner was abusive, for example. However, you would never know that, because outwardly she was completely cheerful. Her face was always glowing like she was in heaven. You would never think there was anything lacking in her life. But she left her parents and siblings when she was a teenager and moved away to another country. With no one to call her own, she lived in a domestic situation that was abusive. She was raising a family in this environment. However, she was never depressed, even for a moment. She was always cheerful and always finding a way out of each single predicament that presented itself. The idea was to be happy for today, and tomorrow will come when it will come. Worrying about it will only ruin today's happiness.

This example does not advocate that someone should stay in an abusive relationship but points out that there are some people out there who can take such a relationship and make something positive out of it. They are the superpeople of the planet and are exceptions from whom we can learn how to take on life.

Which of these two individuals would you rather be? Most people meet a person like the first individual and come out of such a meeting thinking, *Wealth and stature—that is where I want to be.* How about internal happiness? The most common thinking on that is, *Happiness doesn't put food on the table.* However, if you have equanimity, then you can figure out a way to achieve anything. It is the calm and controlled mind that can find its way out of anything. When emotions are introduced, they produce vortices in the mind that make thinking difficult. Fear is the worst emotion. It is entirely suffocating to anything productive. It is fear that destroys all intelligence. People become incapacitated when fear is introduced into any situation.

Therefore, it is important to understand the principles by which fear can be eliminated. There are many ways of reducing the emotional impact of fear. The first exercise that can be carried out is writing. First, make a list of all the things that you are worried about. Now ask yourself, "What is the worst thing that can happen if this worry came true?" Write the answer down. Now, what if it didn't happen? What is the positive counterpart event that could happen? You should observe caution when doing this exercise. Do not list items that are catastrophic in nature, like issues involving life, death, or accident. This exercise is very powerful and should be used with some judicious choosing of items that you need to face. It would be good to do this with a trained professional, such as a yoga therapist.

Now that you have gotten your fears out of your mind, start focusing on the positive aspect of what you want to happen. Take another sheet of paper and write down what you want to happen. Then focus on that. Write out three sentences that would happen as a result of the positive outcome. How would you feel? How would you act? What would you be thinking about?

Now, every morning, take a sheet of paper and write down the outcome that you want to happen and repeat the exercise of how you would feel after that outcome. Also, write down whatever else you think would be associated with that outcome. After every such writing exercise, perform a breathing exercise. The breathing exercise is carried out as follows:

1. Sit down with head, neck, and spine in one line.

2. Relax your shoulders.

3. Make sure there is no tension anywhere in your body.

4. Keep your eyes closed throughout the exercise.

5. Inhale deeply and expand your stomach like a balloon.

6. Exhale completely and let the stomach go deep inside.

7. Repeat the above breathing pattern nine times.

8. Ensure during each cycle that your head, neck, and spine are in one line and your shoulders are relaxed.

Breathing exercises should be carried out each morning to relax the body and, subsequently, the mind.

What would it take to be happy? What would you need to have in your life? Make a list. Look at each item. Focus on the positive every morning. Write out what you would need to make yourself happy and leave the details out. But be sure to act out the feeling of already having obtained that. That is the key. Make that feeling something you wake up for every morning. Have this mini date with yourself every day to reinforce that idea. A possibility only exists when you believe it does. That is the secret. Believe, believe, and believe some more. That is the only way to take the steps to achieve what you want. It is possible. Do leave room for prayer, and feel that a presence is with you that can make it happen. Writing everything down makes us believe it can happen. We need to create the feeling of actually having it in our hands. So the writing exercise should include how the world around us would change.

Here is an example. Let's say you need more money. First, decide how much exactly. Then write down every morning that you make that money, somehow. Write it down as specifically as possible: "I make five thousand dollars a month." Then what would the rest of your world look like, if that came true? You would have a new car. See that in the driveway. You would be a member of tennis or golf groups. You would have the trainers and teachers that you always wanted to have. You would have friends in the upper slices of society. You would have a nice house in a wealthy neighborhood. You would be happy, because you would have all the things you wanted. Have you seen yourself in this detail? You wouldn't have a worried look about being able to pay the bills each month; they would be automatically paid on time. You might plan an elaborate vacation.

See yourself as happy. It will happen. The feeling of happiness brings about a mental state in which possibilities exist. That is the key to life. When you get fearful or angry, it reduces the amount of energy available to you to bring about what you want out of life. The key is not to give in.

There are many examples of people who have survived great odds to achieve what they perceived as success. A successful Ottawa entrepreneur always talks about his hard times starting out. Today he makes a six-figure salary. The key is to have an idea about what you want and don't swerve from it. Show some mettle. If you can't do it yourself, enlist someone who will help you stay on the path to your goal. We very often have great resolve, but we swerve from the goal because we get interested in something else. While it is true that you should be flexible, don't give up on the big picture. If your goal, for example, is to be a successful entrepreneur offering a product to your society, then stay on that path. If other opportunities arise, then you have to review them for how they line up with your original goal. You have to be clear and positive. Always keep that goal in front of you. None of this says that the path is easy. We need to evolve, and therefore, challenges will arise. However, you must consider them as an ocean to cross and pray to be able to cross it. The means and the opportunity to cross will arise. It may take time. Take all the time you need. In the higher world and the bigger picture, time is not as important as the importance we give it. We mistakenly give time and money a disproportionate amount of importance. This needs to be changed, and we need to reassess their place.

Why do we always turn to the hard-luck-turned-good stories? It is because we know we can do it, too. However, we always need to hear it from the outside. It gives us the courage to try it out ourselves. We think, *If they can do it, then probably so can I.* One day I was walking from the bus stop to my destination, which was a ten-minute walk. The wind chill made the temperature -35°C. I was wearing a sari and my legs were cold. On top of that, my hood kept falling off my head because of the wind. So I had to hold my bag of books and my hood and try not to trip because the wind was wrapping the sari around my legs. Throughout that ten-minute walk, I thought of only one thing. I remembered that when I was a child, my mother would walk every day to the local grocery store and walk back with a full bag of groceries. The walk would be fifteen minutes each way, and there was no temperature that would stop her from doing that. She would be dressed in a sari on those trips, as she always was. There was no wearing thermal underwear in those days, either. There was a family of six to feed, including four hungry kids, when she got home. There was no other way to bring the food home each day. So she resolved to go every day no matter what. I remembered her and walked those ten minutes, thinking, *I am doing this out of choice and yet when she walked, she had no choice.* That is an amazing story and it took me to my destination smiling in -35°C weather! It is important to think of amazing stories because they are what help us to cross those oceans of challenges and take us to the shore.

Building an image of you is a very good exercise to get yourself out of a mind-set of only wishing and making it a reality. Once you see a description of the way you want yourself to be, it does not seem like something impossible to do.

# MENTAL FITNESS TRAINING

Fitness professionals spend a lot of time devising techniques for physical fitness. The need for physical fitness is obvious to many in society. Therefore, there are many ways of achieving physical fitness. The goal is to make sure that everyone has some way that they like for keeping fit. Indeed, even the same activity has to be varied to suit the physical needs of the person involved. Each person makes advances in his or her physical ability differently. This must be addressed in prescribing any physical fitness program. This is the strategy used by personal trainers who require detailed physical histories before prescribing the appropriate training schedule. For those who are not active, small amounts of activity are introduced into their lives, so that they will feel a physical change that is suited to them without creating injuries. In the case of an inactive adult, it is more important to get the body comfortable with exercise. In particular, a trainer would be sure to introduce flexibility training. In fact, flexibility training, if introduced into everyone's life at some level, would ward off injuries significantly. Consider daily activities like lifting boxes off the floor. It is easy to hurt the back during such an action. This type of injury would put a person out for a week from regular work and leisure activities, for sure. However, if flexibility training had been introduced in the form of simple stretching, then the individual would know how to carry out the lifting in a safer way.

This is specifically true in the workplace. Most people are in a tense sitting position for eight to ten hours a day. This is bad for the physical body. We need to stretch at regular intervals throughout the day. Bad physical sitting position is responsible for most employee absenteeism. In addition, chronic back and neck pain is common in such an office environment. It is mandatory to introduce stretching into this environment. This stretch break will increase employee effectiveness into the day. Mentally, they will feel refreshed as well.

The more active individual needs to incorporate flexibility training as well. In fact, tightness of the muscles will ensue if flexibility or stretching is not introduced into the training program. An active individual will most likely already incorporate cardiovascular training as well as resistance training into his or her fitness routine. At the level of fitness of an advanced individual, resistance training demands a high level of competence in order to see changes in a body. Therefore, it is all the more necessary in this case to also make sure a regular stretching program is carried out. Otherwise, the muscles do not react in a beneficial way to the physical body. They, instead, get tight and produce cramps, making further training impossible. This leads to lost days in the training schedule.

It is also necessary to mentally prepare for physical training. Mental toughness is increased by sticking to a rigorous and demanding fitness program. We can see this most clearly in the case of marathon runners. Many marathon participants don't look like they could run 26.2 miles; however, it is their mental determination that enables them to finish. In fact, training under inclement conditions gives people the mental toughness advantage that they crave. This is one of the reasons all-weather runners keep up their training. There is nothing quite like the mental gains achieved from running in a winter wind chill of -32°C. It really does make a person feel like she can do anything.

## USING THE BODY-MIND CONNECTION

We have established that there is definitely a mind-body connection. The physical body reacts on the mind. The mind reacts on the body. Just as a rigorous physical training schedule disciplines the mind, mental training techniques can be introduced to discipline the body. The mind-body connection is well known to yoga practitioners. In this ancient science, physical advances are accomplished by mental toughness training. The mind-body connection is further established through breathing. When people are in a state of panic, establishing rhythmical breathing can calm them down. They can then handle the crisis in a more efficient way.

Therefore, breathing properly is not just for physical training. It also creates a calmer mental state. In fact, one way of making progress in meditation is through carrying out a breathing practice, which lasts long enough to ensure the mind is able to focus on its object of meditation. The mind is usually in a state of turmoil incorporating mental vortices. The goal is to pacify those mental vortices through proper mental training techniques. Breathing is one way to calm down the mind. It also has physical benefits. It is known that cardiovascular ability is a function of the nature of one's breathing. The rate and depth of each inhalation is a natural indication of physical health. To illustrate this body-mind connection through breathing, we can use this simple technique of breathing every day for five minutes. Try this simple technique: Sit in a chair with head, neck, and spine in one line. Close your eyes. Inhale and expand your stomach like a balloon. Exhale and let it go deep inside. Repeat nine times. Focus during each breath on yourself and don't let your mind wander to anything else.

More complicated breathing techniques exist; however, they all have limiting populations and cannot be recommended in a general discussion. In fact, if at least one breathing practice is repeated each day, it will naturally calm the mind.

Another mental training technique is focused reading. We generally read in a lazy way. Our minds wander. However, suppose we read in a more determined way. One such method is speed-reading. Read as fast as possible for a designated amount of time. Try to get the salient points. A second way is to memorize. Make sure you choose an uplifting and inspiring piece to memorize. Otherwise, garbage is what you will fill your mind with. Remember always: what your mind is full of is what determines who you are at any given time.

Therefore, choose an inspiring piece to memorize. Start slowly. Memorize three sentences the first day. See if you can remember them that night as well. The whole week, keep up the practice of memorizing three new sentences and trying to recall them at night. The following week increase it by another sentence each week. Build up how much you can memorize at once to a paragraph, and stick with that for six weeks. Then increase again the amount memorized by three sentences a week until you achieve a page. You can stop there and continue memorizing a page a day of an inspirational work for the rest of your life. This is your mental training workout. Just like your physical workout, you need to remain devoted to your mental training workout. It is a marvelous remedy for depression. Depression is a chaotic state of mental panic. Basically your mind is gripped with fear and becomes paralyzed by that state. Mental training techniques unravel the fear and make a person more easily able to think through difficulties. A calmer state of mind is achieved. The combination of breathing and memorization produces a strong mind. Mental toughness creates physical toughness as well. A person is less prone to disease or weakness. A strong body is therefore able to get through the issues of the day.

Writing is yet another wonderful mental training technique. Anger and fear are what prevent us from being happy. Writing is a great therapeutic technique for resolving our anger and fear. Both of these emotions are really the obverse and reverse of the same coin. Fear is generally the cause of all negative emotions. Try taking out a sheet of paper and writing down what is causing your anxiety at any given time. Write it all out. Face it and look at it. It is not necessary that you come up with a solution to the fear. Just writing it out has amazing therapeutic value.

Then let's suppose you could write your dream life. How would you feel? How would you look? What is a typical day for you? Who do you talk to every day? What do you accomplish each day? How do you improve that? Write out everything.

Make a daily list of things to do. This is absolutely necessary. Things magically get accomplished when they are written down. This is miraculous. The mind finds ways to get accomplished those things that it sees written down. Write out your bank balance in your checkbook, if that is part of your goal. Watch it come true. Relax, most importantly. Don't start to feel anxious about your activities. Relax and breathe.

Relaxing also sets things in motion that would not normally be perceived as possible. Let's understand what this relaxation is all about. Does it mean not caring? Does it mean a laissez-faire attitude? It actually means not feeling an emotional connection to the things of the world. When we put emotion into some issue for a certain outcome, we are pulling the forces of the universe into a tug-of-war with us. On the other hand, if we quietly request that it would be to our liking if a certain outcome came about, and then we write it down as something we would like to see happen, then it will probably come to bear in its own natural timeline. By relaxing and letting it go if it is in our best interests, we bring the best to us. It may be that what we want is actually bad for us in the long run. Detachment brings good to us.

Letting go is a really hard exercise to learn. There are many things involved in this. First, we all pin our usefulness to society on someone needing us. It is emotionally hard for us to learn that we are serving a purpose. When that purpose no longer serves us, we will be placed elsewhere. However, this involves giving up our own determined efforts to those of a universal power. What is this universal power? It is that which guides us in a loving way for our own good. When something doesn't work, it is a sign that must be accepted. This is the second difficult lesson for us to learn. We think we know it all. Our ego prevents us from seeing that we could not possibly know it all. We have to surrender for our greater good.

I was training a high-profile person in society at one time. I didn't like the person's attitude toward training, and I had a feeling of incompatibility with the person. I also thought that person was not ready for real training in my style. Circumstances came about that the client could not continue. I desperately thought I had lost someone who would have been very good to train for image purposes alone; however, the universe was not going to allow me to waste my energy on something that was not good for me. It turns out that that client had a lot of anger that was being suppressed. She was trying to understand many things in life and yoga. It was a good choice to ask me to train her; however, that was all she could handle, and more would be counterproductive to her. Sometimes the glamour of the moment prevents us from seeing reality.

# Recommended Training Programs

We need to understand what proper training programs we can use to increase our productivity. Just like our physical training program makes the body into a more efficient machine, mental and spiritual training programs make the human being more effective throughout the day. Creativity is important for problem solving. We encounter many unforeseen events in our day-to-day activities. Some require urgent attention, and some are less sensitive to the decision-making process.

The first thing, then, is to make sure your physical training program accurately reflects who you are and how you operate in life. It needs to be tailored to you. It must give you adequate energy to function throughout your day. It must feed into making you feel mentally refreshed. The body and mind act on each other. Therefore, any physical activity should translate into a good thing for the mind as well. If your physical training program leaves you feeling mentally drained, then it is time to get your physical training program suitably adjusted.

A very common mistake is to fill each day of the week with an activity that absolutely must be carried out, in order to build up an appropriate training program. Using Shanti Consulting's Shantiflex, the same activity stream can be programmed into the client's week in a more appropriate format. The rule for using seven days of the week for training is based on the relative ease of ensuring that the training gets completed within the seven days. It just makes it easy to use. What is special about seven days? How does the body relate to seven days? There is absolutely no relationship. The body has its own natural time scale. It is different for each person. The goal of the personal trainer is now more enhanced. It is his or her job to determine what the most efficient natural time scale would be for each person. An easy way to do this is to start with the seven-day model and then include extra days in between workouts if the person is feeling less rejuvenated. The day in between can be a stretch day. This is the Shantiflex model.

Let's take the example of a runner training for a race. Suppose she has to put thirty to forty miles into her Shantiflex week. This "week" doesn't have to span seven days. In fact, in seven days she would have to put in a lot of miles. Time is an issue. Let's include an extra day or two in the week and use those for stretching. Case histories have shown this to be more effective. Clients were then more effective during their training runs. Not only does this give the body a better chance to recover, but it also gives the body time to stretch. Stretching is a much-needed activity, but we don't program in enough time to stretch. We should stretch every day. We should stretch after each and every physical activity. For example, we need to stretch after every weight-training or resistance-training session. We should not stretch before the session, since we might make the muscle easily supple enough to tear during a heavy load. This is a topic of much debate in the academic human kinetics world. Stretching is also a mental exercise. It delivers a message to your body that you care enough to take care of it. You're not constantly abusing and disciplining your body. You love it and want to take care of it. This is an important exercise.

Most people who engage in an exercise program start off disliking their bodies. Their bodies sense that and deliver depression to their minds. They start off on an exercise program and find they are not mentally feeling any better. They feel worse. This can be offset by the endorphins released during exercise; however, this feeling is short-lived. Stretching puts back the feeling of love and doesn't make the body feel strained. The body generally feels strained for two reasons: either we experience a physical strain from purely physical activity or we experience mental strain, which is also reflected in a sore body. Mental strain is stress or fear that is introduced into the mind, which finds its way into the body. Stretching is private time with your body. Studies have shown that people who stretch have fewer injuries and less mental stress. Somehow spending care time with your body also slows you down enough not to worry and to care for the most important thing you own: your body. Each stretch needs to be held for twenty to thirty seconds. During this time, your mind gets slowed down. Of course, it will wander to things you are most worried about. The trick is to get the mind back to focusing on the stretch. This is an amazing meditation and cannot be underestimated as a tool for clarifying thoughts.

We are normally afraid because we typically think of only one outcome for a certain event. We focus on only that outcome, and it becomes a reality for us in our minds. We throw our whole body-mind system completely out of whack based on that hypothetical result. Instead, we need to theoretically accept the fact that there are many possible outcomes for any sequence of events. During quiet time, we can afford to think of alternate outcomes. We can dream of what we wish to occur. Let us give ourselves permission to dream for that brief amount of time. It helps to expand our vision, and for that time, we will not feel afraid. This has great therapeutic benefits for the mind and the body. Letting ourselves feel good is an excellent exercise.

Most people find that food helps them do this; however, our society is becoming obese because many people turn to food as a narcotic for allowing themselves to forget. The inside strength is so gripping that they can only find escape through gross physical pleasure.

Deliberately tuning out the outside world and focusing on you is the key to happiness. Fear ensues because we focus on the outside world. We need to focus on ourselves. Stretching is a first step to establishing meditation. Reading anything uplifting is another technique for disciplining the mind. Memorization techniques were previously discussed. However, just getting into the practice of reading is an excellent way to keep the mind vibrant. It is difficult to explain how ideas come into the mind; however, if we keep ourselves open to the muse by reading other people's works, it becomes easier for that force to help us as well. Ideas are the way we survive. We don't give enough value to or put enough emphasis on them as a society. How else do you get through the day?

No day goes by on autopilot. We are here because our ancestors were ingenious. Our families depend on our ingenuity. Alternately, we grow through the development of ideas. Have you ever gone through a week and not had an original thought? Don't you feel tired? It is because you have given in to a morbid state of routine. Never get into that. It is like being brain dead, and it makes you feel like a zombie. We need to constantly feel invigorated. That is why the human brain is larger than that of any other species on the planet. We have evolved a giant brain. We need to use it. Use it or lose it. The moment you feel like you are on autopilot, head to your local library and check out a book—any book will do for emergencies—and then read it. Even write a summary of it at the end for your own good. You may pass it on to someone else who has an interest in the book. There is a magical thing that occurs when you read a book. The ideas of the author that are floating in that space have come to your space and you are now co-living with that author, who does not necessarily need to be alive.

Have you ever seen a movie and later thought unconsciously about the actors in that movie? Do you think to yourself, *I wonder what so-and-so is doing these days*? You are living with the actor's psyche. Of course, this gets brushed off in a day or two, and the effect is gone. However, we have been touched in a small way by the effect of the movie. Similarly, this effect is apparent in books. Some people speed-read. In this way, they have forced their minds to live with the author for an intense burst. The effect is the same; however, you do get the gist of the work faster. That is the way speed-reading works.

Similarly, you can start on a writing exercise program. Suppose you wrote each day. Get up in the morning and write a page on anything. It is amazing how this kick-starts your day. It is better than coffee. It actually helps you be more alert during the day. Try this exercise for a period of four weeks and feel the mental effects. Writing is an amazing mental training technique. It can cure depression.

Depression is caused by a disorganized mental state. The mind can't see a way out of its problems. It is usually full of fear. Suppose we again used the medium of writing to propose other ways out. Suppose we just wrote down "There is a way out." Suppose we got up each morning and wrote down, "There is a way out" about ten times each day. Then we filled the rest of the page with random thoughts. We can explain our predicament. This helps to vent as well. We can vent our anger. It will definitely change our personality. Vent on paper. Vent everything like hopes, dreams, fears, and anger. Anger is actually an extreme form of fear. Know that, if you have anger, it is because you did not resolve your fear when it was in the stage of fear. You let it grow into a weed of anger with big roots. You need to ferret out, from your writing, the real cause of your anger. What or who is it that you need to address? Don't worry about finding an answer today. It will definitely come. Be patient.

Meditation is an excellent tool for mental training; however, it requires patience. The first time you try meditation, it feels horrible. But in fact, that is when the most work is being done. All the thoughts that come to you during quiet time are what you really need to pay attention to. Persevere. Choose a lofty statement that can inspire you. Repeat it silently to yourself. When other thoughts come, mentally note what you are worried about. It is your mind talking to you. Once you note what you are being presented with, over the course of time, those thoughts will not bother you. You can start your first meditation session with five minutes. A lot of distractions will come. You can note all the things you are worried about and then continue on. It is like the first time you ever set about to work out. You think about all the things you probably should be doing. It is amazing what kind of excuses you give yourself. Some of them are quite comical. But we need to persevere. A lot of benefit comes from meditation. It is good to meditate first thing in the morning and when you come home from work in the evening. This helps clear the flood of emotions from the workday and gives you a clean slate into your evening hours. You may also come up with ideas for the next day's events. It is important to see what you are thinking about. Continue to meditate and see what influence this has on your mind-body system. Your body will react to this meditation in a favorable way. It will feel more relaxed. Physical strain is related to the mental barrage of thoughts that lay hidden in the mind space. They make your body feel strained. A stretch session is absolutely mandatory if you want relief from this cycle.

# Conclusions

If we are to survive in this world with its day-to-day experiences, then we must align ourselves with who we really are. From that standpoint, we will be better able to generate honest happiness in the face of any circumstances. If we truly want to feel independent of the sway of the climate of the emotions around us, we need to be honest and decide who we really are. From that standpoint, we can always decide if an action is good for us or not. If we constantly turn our face outside, we will never be in alignment with our true self. In those cases, we suffer. In our interactions with others, we must always fall back on our honest self. Otherwise, the mind games can destroy us. Outguessing others or the outside world is the surest recipe for disaster. True happiness and efficiency in action with the outside world comes from being authentic. Find out who you really are. When you focus on yourself, your actions reveal that honesty. Revel in who you are and celebrate it. This is the true secret.

We have discussed many ways to generate that honesty. First, it is important to develop a physical fitness program with a professional trainer. Remember that your body, mind, and spirit are linked. Therefore, any changes in your physical being will affect your mind and spirit as well. These changes will also transform your outlook. Problem solving can be influenced through this method of physical fitness training. With the advice of a professional trainer, it is possible to devise a program that will be of interest to you. This is the key. Professionals know what works for you and can develop an individualized program for you. This exercise program can take many forms. It can include traditional cardiovascular activity, resistance training, and stretching. Using the unique Shantiflex program, you can train in a way that is pain free but makes the gains you need to see progress. This is the benefit of Shantiflex, which enables your workout program to be spread out over more than a week and according to your lifestyle.

Breathing is a great tool for clearing your mind. It aligns the whole body's processes and makes it more efficient at everything. In fact, if you just did breathing exercises, you would be amazed at how much calmer you will feel. Simple breathing can have amazing results. At any given time during the day, it is how you breathe that determines your mental and physical state of mind. Indeed, that can be changed by breathing properly. This is the secret. When we are angry or frustrated, our breath is shallow and quick. When we are calm, like lying on a beach, our breath is more deep and relaxed. This is the natural state. If we practiced regular breathing exercises, we would make a change in how we naturally breathe. This, in turn, changes how we think. Our decision-making processes are better, naturally. We are calmer and can make decisions at a better level of thinking. We are not gripped and paralyzed by fear. We are aware of our alternatives, and therefore, our decision making is better. Breathing can change the way you feel. Next time your nerves are getting to you, try a simple breathing exercise for five minutes. Then see how the world around you changes. It is truly an amazing tool.

Stretching is another way of getting a handle on our body, mind, and spirit combination. Stretching gives us time to slow down. Each stretch has to be held for twenty seconds. During that time, we are automatically slowed down. Yoga has similar parallels and can be a form of stretching as well. In yoga, however, our breathing must be synchronized with our motions. In addition, we make our mind so focused that it can think of the infinite during the time we are in the yoga asana, or position. Practicing yoga for fifteen minutes a day makes us feel like we can accomplish anything. It calms us down, and we are physically stronger.

Second, you need to address your mental space. Think of starting by reading. Read a variety of books. Both fiction and nonfiction are acceptable. Too many times, we stay within our comfort zones and are afraid to venture out. We need to expand our thinking horizon if we are to make gains in our problem-solving ability. Reading biographies helps people to become inspired. Sometimes this takes the form of "If they did it, then so can I." Sometimes that is enough to get someone out of a stuck position. The person just needed a mental jolt to get unstuck. Reading a variety of books helps keep us on the plane of reality and generates ideas in the idea space.

Third, we need to write. Writing makes our nerve currents active and generates ideas. We may see our way out of a difficult problem by the mere fact of writing out the problem. Write for three pages each morning. This activity is designed to kick-start the nerve currents in your brain so that your thinking is better. The first page will be safe territory. You may write down your to-do list or the anticipated outcomes of meetings you have during the day. On the second page is where fun starts. You really have to bring out of yourself the stuff that you didn't want to see on paper. But you need to see it to face it. In addition, you can write down problems that you don't see solutions to; this method can help produce a solution to your problem. This occurs just from the mere fact of writing it down. It is truly an amazing and underutilized tool. If everyone wrote three pages in the morning, the world would be a better place. Problem solving would be easier if we practiced this exercise every morning.

In addition, writing is a great tool to alleviate anger. Writing out your anger does seem like a big relief. It releases the pent-up energy that you hide. This pent-up energy is useful energy that is inside you but is wasting you away. It prevents you from thinking straight. Therefore, you need to alleviate this block by writing it down. Just write. Don't ask how. There is no need to stick to any form where emotions are involved. You simply need to get the energy out of yourself by writing. You will be amazed at how much better you feel.

Finally, meditation is another tool to use to get control of our body, mind, and spirit. The meaning of the word *meditation* is "to measure the mind." During meditation, you are measuring the mind's contents. Sitting quietly, you repeat an uplifting line. Something like "I am important to me" can be used. While saying that statement to yourself, other thoughts come and interrupt. You must note them and move on. Don't pay any attention to dealing with those thoughts at the time of meditation. Just note them, write them down on a piece of paper, and go back to the repetition. It is important to do this for the full fifteen minutes. Otherwise, your mind fools itself and thinks it is quite fine. In reality, a lot of turmoil is going on, and you need to give those thoughts a chance to surface. Definitely in fifteen minutes, they will surface. Just noting that they are there is actually enough; you need not spend time agonizing over solutions. They will resolve themselves. They could be part of the next day's writing exercise. Being aware of your attitudes is half the battle in dealing with the outside world. Your actions at any given time are a product of your thoughts; therefore, if you want your actions to be the correct ones for you, then you really need to spend time understanding what your mind is filled with. It could be a true revelation that something really is bothering you. However, if you don't take the time to identify it, then it comes up at the most inappropriate time and starts to interfere with your daily work. For example, you may find yourself getting angry at the wrong person. This is obviously the mind's way of dealing with something in a safe way. In actuality, it is a bad way of dealing with the issue. Obviously you need to deal with it at the level at which it is occurring. You may have to confront the person you are angry with. Or resolve it in your own mind that you are not really angry at the person but instead are afraid of a consequence of some action. That is a different problem. However, you would not be aware of this circumstance unless you had carried out the meditation session. This is the secret.

In summary, we need to address the integration of our body, mind, and spirit in order to behave effectively with the outside world. We need to spend time developing that integration so that we can be naturally more effective in all our activities. However, just like an athlete who must practice every day, we must also train ourselves in some way each day to develop an attitude that makes us effective. We must examine ourselves and develop a constructive training program. This program must address the body, mind, and spirit. Fitness is not just about the body. It is about our integrated system. Mental and spiritual fitness is equally important. If they are not addressed, our physical fitness alone will not carry us through the demanding lifestyles that we all lead.

It is my prayer that the information in this book can be used by many people to become more effective in this world.

# About the Author

Hema holds a PhD in aerospace engineering from the University of Toronto. She is listed in *Who's Who in the World*, and she is a yoga instructor, personal trainer, and expert in East Indian philosophy. Hema has a keen interest in training the complete being rather than just the physical body. She is a canfitpro PTS (Personal Trainer Specialist), kettlebell, and TRX (Total Resistance Exercise) certified instructor and has undergone intensive training in India at the Swami Vivekananda Yoga Research Institute (SVYASA, an esteemed university). Hema is a regular Sanskrit instructor for Samskrita Bharati, having conducted a camp for yoga instructors. She completed an advanced degree in yoga philosophy and Sanskrit from Karnataka State Open University, India, and has published in India's leading yoga philosophy journal, *Prabuddha Bharata*. She has also completed an advanced yoga therapy course with Svastha Yoga. Hema regularly gives workshops on wellness to workplaces in the Ottawa area and is a regular presenter at fitness conferences. Hema is currently an engineering consultant at Shanti Engineering and Research.